EVERYTHING YOU NEED TO KNOW ABOUT YOUR EYES

Everything you need to know about your eyes

DR ROBERT YOUNGSON
MB., ChB., D.O.

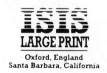

ISIS
LARGE PRINT
Oxford, England
Santa Barbara, California

Copyright © R.M. Youngson 1985
First published in Great Britain 1985 by Sheldon
Press, SPCK, Marylebone Road, London NW1 4DU

Published in Large print 1990 by Clio Press,
55 St. Thomas' Street, Oxford OX1 1JG,
by arrangement with Sheldon Press

British Libary Cataloguing in Publication Data
Youngson, R. M. (Robert Murdoch), 1926 –
Everything you need to know about your eyes.
1. Man. Eyes. Diseases
I. Title
617.7

ISBN 1-85089-395 0

Printed and bound by Hartnolls Ltd.,
Bodmin, Cornwall
Cover designed by CGS Studios, Cheltenham

Contents

Preface

Many people, especially as they grow older, worry about their eyes and their vision. I know, because it is my job to conserve sight and a very important part of my work to encourage people to tell me exactly what they are anxious about so that I can reassure them that a good deal of the worry is unnecessary. Very often it results from a lack of understanding of what causes difficulty in reading or seeing TV, blurring or fogging of vision, aches and pains, and so on.

So in this book I hope to do two things. First, to provide an easily understood and comforting explanation of many common eye symptoms. Second, to draw attention to those eye problems which do need expert specialist attention and which, in most cases, can be treated effectively.

Dr Robert Youngson, 1985

The eye

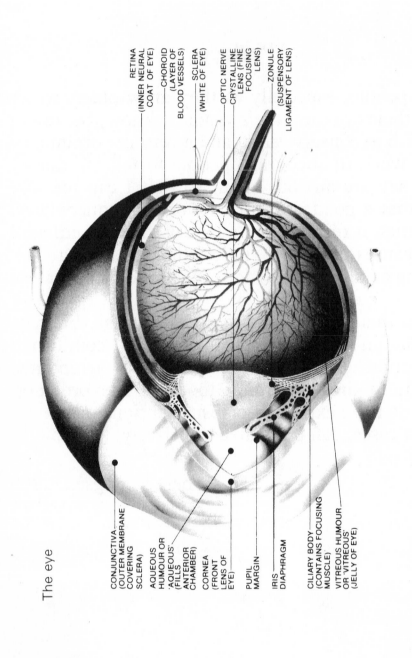

CONJUNCTIVA
(OUTER MEMBRANE
COVERING
SCLERA)

AQUEOUS
HUMOUR OR
'AQUEOUS'
(FILLS
ANTERIOR
CHAMBER)

CORNEA
(FRONT
LENS OF
EYE)

PUPIL
MARGIN

IRIS
DIAPHRAGM

CILIARY BODY
(CONTAINS FOCUSING
MUSCLE)

VITREOUS HUMOUR
OR 'VITREOUS'
(JELLY OF EYE)

RETINA
(INNER NEURAL
COAT OF EYE)

CHOROID
(LAYER OF
BLOOD VESSELS)

SCLERA
(WHITE OF EYE)

OPTIC NERVE

CRYSTALLINE
LENS (FINE
FOCUSING
LENS)

ZONULE
(SUSPENSORY
LIGAMENT OF LENS)

CHAPTER
ONE

Who Needs Glasses?

One thing I want to make perfectly plain: the purpose of glasses is to enable you to see properly, and that's all. If you can see clearly without glasses, you don't need them and shouldn't wear them. There is no such thing as "eye-strain"; even if your vision without glasses is very poor and you persistently try to see without glasses, you will do yourself no harm. You might feel discomfort or give yourself a headache by prolonged screwing-up of your eyes, but you will not damage them. So, in adults, glasses are simply prescribed to enable you to see better.

The only exception occurs in children below the age of eight. From birth to about eight, the eyes and the brain continue to develop and it is essential for the full, normal development of the visual system that children should have clear vision in both eyes. Eye doctors are especially concerned about this and stress the importance of children wearing their prescribed glasses constantly. But so far as the health of your eyes is concerned, from the age of about eight onwards, it simply doesn't matter whether you wear glasses or not.

Presbyopia

If you are over forty-five, you probably have this, although you may not be aware of it and it should not alarm you. Like most medical terms, the name comes from Greek: presbus meaning "an old man" and presbyopia "old man's vision".

Presbyopia is the condition in which you find that you need to hold your book or paper further and further away from your eyes, in order to see the print clearly. Usually, the early stages pass unnoticed, because the process is very gradual, and it may be quite some time before you notice that anything is amiss. Often, the first sign occurs when you try to make out small print in a poor light and find that the letters are too small to be resolved.

To be accurate, presbyopia is simply the latter stage of a process which has been going on from early childhood. You may have observed children reading with their noses about two inches away from the book. They do so because they like to see the print as large a possible and they have not the slightest difficulty in focusing their eyes at such a short range. They see the print very clearly and easily and there is absolutely no harm in their reading this way. Indeed, to do so effectively exercises the convergence (turning in of the eyes) which is a very good thing. But if you watch a teenager, with normal vision, reading a book, you will see that it is held further away. People in their twenties and thirties will usually hold books on their laps, when reading, and those in their forties will almost always do so. This is perfectly normal.

Older people, who read with the print close to their eyes are "short-sighted", that is, they can't see clearly at a distance. Round about forty-five, people who have never had problems with their vision find that they have to hold books or papers uncomfortably far away and if the print is small, the effect of perspective may make it difficult or impossible to read. It is interesting to appreciate that this process would be very much less obvious were it not that reading is so important to us and that, for reasons of economy and/or convenience, print has to be reasonably small. The problem shows itself when the nearest point at which we can focus becomes so far away from our eyes that normal print cannot be read clearly. Anyone with presbyopia can, if they wish, go on reading for a year or two longer without glasses, by borrowing large-print books from the library.

Many presbyopes tell me that the problem is worse in the evenings and suggest that this is perhaps because they are tired. In fact, the problem is much reduced by bright light and as daylight is much brighter than artificial lighting, this is why they have more trouble at night. A good reading light positioned close to the book will reflect so much light into your eyes that the pupils may become almost as small as they are in daylight, and it is the smallness of the pupils that increases the depth of focus, in the same way that "stopping down" a camera iris diaphragm does. I want to stress that presbyopia is *not* a disease. It is perfectly natural, and eventually affects all of us. You will find it helpful in understanding what happens if you look at the diagram of the eye

3

(facing page 1) before reading on.

The human eye closely resembles a television camera: both have a lens system, with a mechanism for regulating the amount of light allowed to enter (the iris diaphragm) and a screen at the back on which an image is thrown by the lens. The main lens of the eye, the cornea, which is kept wet and clean by a regular but unnoticed production of tears and the wiping action of the eyelids, does most of the bending of the light necessary to form the image of whatever one is looking at. But there is a second, less powerful crystalline lens, lying immediately behind the iris, that allows the eye to change focus. With the inner lens in its thinnest condition, the eye is in focus for distant objects, and if we wish to see near things clearly, the crystalline lens changes its shape and becomes thicker, in order to bend the light rays more. Knowing how it does this will enable you to understand how presbyopia occurs.

The adjustable crystalline lens is supported by an attached collar of fibres around its edge and it is these fibres (called zonules) that exert a pull on the edge to increase the diameter of the lens and make it thinner from front to back, as necessary. In childhood and youth, the lens is very elastic, and as soon as the pull on the fibres is relaxed, the lens will become thicker and more curved. The supporting collar of the lens is attached in its turn to an outer ring of focusing muscle. When the muscle acts, the ring becomes smaller, releases the tension on the lens and allows it to become more curved, and stronger. When a young person looks at something near, the lenses are so elastic that they easily adjust to the highly curved shape necessary to form a clear image. The name of this unconscious, automatic changing of focus for different distances of viewing is called "accommodation".

The reason why our lenses don't remain elastic all through life is rather curious. The fine, transparent fibres of which the lens is made, are manufactured in the region where the zonules are attached. As they grow, these fibres fit neatly together inside the capsule of the lens to form a perfectly shaped structure. Quite early in childhood, the lenses are complete and working beautifully and if the fibre manufacture were to stop then we would have no problems later. Unfortunately, there is no way to stop the production of ever more of these fibres and the result is that, the older we get, the tighter and less elastic our lenses become. By about the age of sixty, the lenses have become so rigid that they cannot alter the focus of the eyes at all.

Reading glasses

If a person's eyes are capable of perfect focus, for distant objects, with the crystalline lenses relaxed, he will continue to see clearly in the distance and unless some disease or injury occurs, there is no reason why he should not do so indefinitely. However, reading glasses will be needed to enable the eyes to focus on near objects. These have ordinary lenses, known as spheres, of quite weak power — much weaker, for instance, than the cornea, but this power will have to

5

be increased progressively, as the crystalline lenses become less and less able to do the job themselves.

Opticians and eye doctors express the power of spectacle lenses in units called dioptres and the usual prescription for the first pair of reading glasses, at about the age of forty-five, is one dioptre. At fifty, most people will need one and a half dioptres, at fifty-five about two dioptres and at sixty, two and a half. A person with healthy eyes should never need to have a reading addition of more than two and a half dioptres, nor should it be necessary for the reading glasses to be changed more than at five-yearly intervals. So four different prescriptions should cover your life-time requirements for reading glasses. The common habit of urging patients to return to the optician "for a check-up" every two years, is quite unnecessary.

If a sixty-year-old person, with normal distance vision, puts a 1 dioptre lens in front of each eye, he will see clearly an object placed at 1 metre distance. But this is too far away for reading. If he tries 2 dioptre lenses, he will see clearly at half a metre, and 3 dioptre lenses will enable him to see clearly at one third of a metre (one foot) — but this is too near for comfortable reading and would probably cause problems in maintaining alignment of the two eyes. What he wants is a power that will allow clear vision at somewhere between a half and a third of a metre, say about 40 centimetres. Lenses of 2.5 dioptre will do the trick nicely and this is what you will need for reading, at sixty, if your distance vision is normal.

Everything I have written so far is with reference

to normal distance vision. Now we come to the other reasons for wearing glasses.

Myopia (short sight)

Shortsighted people's eyes are naturally in focus for near objects and many of them do not need reading glasses. But this advantage is always offset by poor far-away vision. As they get older short-sighted people have exactly the same progressive loss of lens elasticity as everyone else and, if they are wearing glasses to give them clear distance vision, the progressive difficulty in close work is as apparent to them as anyone else. But as soon as they take off their glasses, they can see clearly at close range and many short-sighted people do remove their glasses for this purpose. I doubt if there is any real harm in this, although it has been suggested that, in the earlier stages of presbyopia, one may be depriving oneself of the chance to exercise whatever focusing one has left. I think this is rather an academic point and not one that anyone should worry about.

The official name for short sight is "myopia", another Greek word, in which "myo" means "muscular" and is a reference to the fact that, before spectacles were invented, the only thing short-sighted people could do to improve distant vision was to screw up their eyes, by using the muscle around the lids. "Muscular vision" doesn't alter the focus of the eyes, but it does increase the depth of field, as already explained.

The onset of myopia

Myopia usually starts at, or around, puberty when body growth takes a spurt, usually progresses along the body growth, and nearly always stops progressing when body growth stops, around the age of twenty-five. It is quite rare for myopia to progress after that age. People in which it does so will usually have become short-sighted early in life and will already be severely myopic by early adult life. In the enormous majority of cases short sight is in no sense a disease.

What happens in myopia is that the eyes grow slightly larger than is appropriate for the focal length of the cornea and crystalline lens, so that the image of the distant object is not focused on the inside back of the eye (the retina) as it should be, but at a point in front. Consequently, when rays of light reach the retina the image is blurred. Rays of light coming from near objects, however, spread out more, when they reach the eye, than those from distant objects, and focus further back, perhaps exactly in the plane of the retina.

So, the lenses in glasses for short sight are of opposite type to those in reading glasses. Short-sight glasses have lenses that are thinner in the middle than at the edges, called minus spheres. Instead of causing light rays to come together, these cause them to spread out, and that is what people need if their eyes cause the rays to focus too soon.

So how important is it for short-sighted young people to wear glasses? In the rare cases of extremely short sight (one in a thousand), vision without glasses will be extremely blurred, even at short ranges, and it is essential for very young children in this situation to wear glasses, if visual development is to be normal. I would not hesitate to prescribe glasses, or even contact lenses, for a baby of eighteen months if I found very severe short sight (or any other defect of focus) at that age. We now recognise that in such rare cases this is the only hope for the development of normal vision in later life. After the age of about eight, glasses will make no difference to the visual development, but will make a great difference to the child's educational progress.

In normal degrees of short sight, the eye-brain system will be mature before short sight shows itself and there will be no advantage on that score. In most cases, elementary education will have been completed also, and the only disadvantage will be the inability to see clearly in the distance. This can cause difficulty in seeing blackboards, watching TV, and recognizing friends across the road (which may lead to social problems). These young people can easily read, without glasses, and often tend to become bookish, because of their dependence on reading for information. So glasses should be worn at all times, and this is the advice usually given.

However, one needs to give due weight to the, sometimes severe, adverse psychological effects of glasses on young people. This is a very variable factor: many seem not to mind at all, but some are deeply distressed and seriously upset. Young people are unimaginatively and, sometimes, unimaginably, cruel to one another in their comments about, and attitudes to, things like the wearing of glasses — and young lives can be made a real misery. In rare instances, the advantages of glasses may be out-weighed by the social and psychological effects, in which case the glasses are justifiably abandoned. I see this problem frequently and know that thousands of teenage myopes often feel themselves in an intolerable position because an optician or eye doctor insists that glasses must be worn and implies that eye damage may result if they are not. I frequently fit quite young people with contact lenses as a way round this problem.

Hypermetropia

This condition is most commonly called "long sight", which gives rise to considerable confusion and misunderstanding. In hypermetropia, the power of the cornea is insufficient so that, if the eye remains in a completely relaxed state, as it ought for distance vision, the rays of light do not come to focus on the retina. The eye is too short for the power of its focusing lens. But, if the person concerned is young enough, he can get things right by accommodation (or focusing) to strengthen the power of the eye so that the image is sharply cast on the retina. Young people have a wonderful range of focusing power, and do this continuously without being aware of it. Indeed, unless it is very severe, hypermetropia is usually discovered in young people only if it causes them to focus so hard that one eye is pulled inwards, causing a squint (see Chapter 5). In other cases the condition is simply not suspected and there is no harm in this. All that happens is that these young people constantly exercise the focusing muscles.

However, as previously explained, the power of focusing falls off steadily, in everyone, with increasing age. A person with neither myopia nor hypermetropia may require reading glasses at about forty-five. But if a degree of focusing (accommodation) is needed even for distance vision, an even stronger effort will be required for closer viewing and the time will inevitably come when the person concerned exhausts his range of accommodation. The effect of this is exactly as if presbyopia were occurring at an earlier age, though this will vary according to the severity of the hypermetropia. A person with mild hypermetropia might need reading glasses at the age of thirty, while, in a severe case, they might be needed in the teens.

At a later stage, even the distance vision is going to be affected by hypermetropia — one reason why the term "long-sight" is not a very good one. Consider the sixty-year-old whose crystalline lenses have, typically, become completely rigid and have no accommodation left. If neither myopic nor hypermetropic, such a person will have clear distance vision. But, if even a small degree of hypermetropia exists, he will have severe blurring both at a distance and near to, for there is nothing he can do to strengthen the lenses of his eyes. He will therefore need glasses for distance and a second pair, 2.50 dioptres stronger, for reading. And that brings us to the question of . . .

11

Bifocals

These can be very convenient and many people swear by them. They come in many different designs, but all have lenses with stronger lower segments. In the bifocals of an elderly person with two and a half dioptres of short sight (ability to see clearly objects close by), the lower segments will be of plain glass.

The segment of the lens intended for reading should be no larger than is necessary for this purpose, because if it takes up more of the spectacle lens, the field of clear vision for distance will be restricted unnecessarily. When reading, one looks only down and in, so the type of bifocal in which the whole bottom half of each lens is of near-vision power, is not really suitable for normal usage. The small semi-circle of extra power, for near sight, set in the lower part of the lens slightly in towards the nose, has been shown, by years of trial and error, usually to be the best. If you don't like the look of this, you might like to consider having "invisible" bifocals and pay the extra cost.

Some people have great difficulty in getting used to bifocals and very often the reason is that the lower segment is too large. We look down, quite naturally not only when reading, but also when walking downstairs or stepping off kerbs. This is the most common problem with bifocals: obviously, if you look through the stronger reading segment when you want to see something further away, as a kerb will be, the object you are looking at will be out of focus. Older people sometimes find this alarming and dangerous until they understand what is happening and learn to adapt. The trick is to turn the head, rather than the eyes, downwards, so that one is looking through the distance part of the lenses.

A convenient form of "bifocal" is the "half-frame" type of spectacles. These are light, comfortable and efficient for those whose distance vision is adequate, and can be worn constantly if desired.

Astigmatism

This is the last of the types of focusing error I have to explain, and the least easy to understand. It is not essential for you to read this section in order to understand the rest of the book and I only include it for the sake of completeness and to satisfy those who prefer to have everything explained.

Again, the name comes from Greek and means "not a spot". An optical system with astigmatism causes unequal magnification of the same object in different directions so, if we are trying to focus a spot of light to form a spot image, an astigmatic lens will produce a kind of blurred line instead. People with astigmatism have corneas that are more egg-shaped than part of a perfect sphere, and an egg-shaped cornea will focus a spot at two different distances, the nearer one corresponding to its steeper curve, and the further one corresponding with its flatter curve. The egg may be on its side, or on its end, or even lying obliquely, so that the "axis" of the astigmatism may be horizontal or vertical or at any oblique angle in between.

People with "pure" astigmatism have corneas which are perfect in focus along one curve (meridian), but either short-sighted or long-sighted in the meridian at right angles. However, most people with astigmatism are either short-sighted in both meridians, long-sighted in both meridians, or have one short-sighted and one long-sighted meridian. Note that the meridians of maximum and minimum curvature are always at right angles to each other.

Lenses to correct astigmatism are called "cylindrical" lenses but most people with astigmatism will need lenses which combine either plus or minus spheres with an appropriate cylinder, set at a proper axis.

Astigmatism is the one type of focusing error in which clear vision can be obtained only by glasses (or contact lenses). The myope can see things clearly without glasses and the young hypermetrope can accommodate. But the astigmat has no such resources. Accommodation can focus one meridian but will put the other further out of focus, and near viewing makes no difference to the basic problem. People with a minor degree of astigmatism don't usually bother about glasses as they will see well enough for most practical purposes. But high astigmats must choose between going about in a constant blur or wearing glasses or contact lenses full-time. Again I would emphsise that, after the age of about eight, no harm will be caused to the eyes by *not* wearing glasses. Astigmats sometimes get a headache from tensing the muscles around the eyes, but there is no way the eyes can be damaged.

Contact lenses

This is much too large a subject to be dealt with here. But, for those who are interested, I have written a book exclusively about contact lenses (*Everthing You Need to Know about Contact Lenses*, Sheldon Press, 1984) which covers the subject thoroughly

Illumination

I have already mentioned that if the pupils of the eyes can be made small ("stopping down") any focusing error can be helped or even, sometimes, eliminated. When the pupils are small, less light gets into the eyes and if, for instance, they were made small by the use of appropriate eye-drops, everything would look very gloomy and dark. But if we made the pupils small by raising the intensity of the light shining on whatever we are looking at, this will not apply and we will benefit from the optical improvements of a stopped-down system. One's natural inclination might be to put stonger wattage bulbs in the sockets and this may help a little, but it is by no means the best way of going about it.

When rays of light travel outwards from a light source, they do so in straight lines and in every direction. If we wanted to capture all the light coming from the source, we would have to surround it by a hollow sphere so that the light would shine only on the inner surface. Imagine a small light at the centre of a sphere of radius 1 metre, that is, where the distance from the light to the inside surface of the sphere is 1 metre. Suppose we measure the brightness of the light at any point on that inner surface and note the figure — say 9 candle-power. Now, imagine the same light at the centre of a larger sphere, of radius 3 metres, so that the surface of the sphere is now three times as far away. The same amount of light now has to spread itself over a surface which is much more than three times that of the smaller sphere. In fact, the surface area of the larger sphere is *nine* times the area of the smaller one and, consequently, the brightness will only be one ninth.

This is called the "inverse square" law. Brightness does not decline in simple proportion to the distance from the light; it declines in proportion to the distance multiplied by itself, that is, the *square* of the distance. If you move a light twice as far away, the brightness will be reduced to one quarter; if you move it three times as far away, the brightness will be reduced to one ninth; if you move it ten times as far away, the brightness will be reduced to one hundredth! This means that a 100 watt bulb at 1 foot distance, produces the same brightness as would a 1000 watt bulb 10 feet away, up in the middle of the ceiling. Even the best artificial lighting is likely to be much less bright than daylight, but here is a way of counterbalancing the fact and giving yourself the benefit of the improved vision to be obtained from small pupils.

So, by far the best type of reading lamp is one which can be adjusted to focus direct light, from a *short* distance on to the book or paper you are reading. Science and fashion seldom take much note of one another, but, in the case of the decorative trend towards multiple table lamps rather than lights in the ceiling, we have an example of a happy coincidence of interests.

Intolerance to glasses

This is very common and is a cause of great annoyance, both to patients and to the opticians who have prescribed or dispensed the glasses. The annoyance, in the case of the latter, is sometimes compounded by the uneasy knowledge that the trouble is of their own making. I don't think this happens very often in the case of experienced and careful practitioners and, indeed, the general standard of optical prescription and dispensing has improved markedly in recent years, but it is undeniable that a good many people do not get the satisfaction and full utility from their glasses that they are entitled to expect.

However, a good deal of apparent intolerance to glasses is due to the presence of eye disease which no lenses can correct. If patients complain that their glasses do not relieve them of glare when looking towards bright lights or, alternatively, do not clear up foggy vision or restore absent vision, there is the possibility of cataract or glaucoma or some other disease of the eyes. In such a case, however, the optician should recognize the presence of such conditions and should not allow the patient to believe, even by implication, that the glasses will cure the defect.

One of the commonest causes of discomfort with

spectacles is poor centring. To explain this important matter, I have to make brief mention of prisms. A prism is a wedge of glass or other transparent material. When one looks through a prism, whatever one is looking at seems to have been moved a little to one side, because the prism bends the light rays, without changing their focus. When a prism is placed in front of one eye there is double vision, but often the eye can move, independently of the other eye, so as to fuse the two images into one. This may, however, involve strain.

I'm not suggesting that opticians deliberately put prisms in people's glasses so they are forced to turn their eyes in or out all the time. But that is what, in effect, happens. If you reverse your spectacles, and move the lenses from side to side while looking through them, you will see that when you look through a lens near the edge, the image is displaced to one side or the other. Any lens may, for this purpose, be considered as a pair of prisms joined, base to base or apex to apex.

So it is of great importance that the lenses in your spectacles should be so placed in the frames that you look through their exact optical centres. If you do not, you will have a prismatic effect and, all the time you are seeing with them, you will have to keep your eyes turned (probably inwards) to avoid double vision. Long-sighted people wearing lenses in frames so large that the lenses cannot be centred, will be wearing "base-out" prisms and, even when looking into the remote distance, will have to keep their eyes turned inwards as if looking at something near. No wonder they feel uncomfortable. And so much for fashionable giant frames!

Proper centring of spectacle lenses demands that the distance between your pupils should be accurately measured, with your eyes aligned on an object at a distance appropriate to the glasses. This means that the inter-pupil distance may have to be measured both when you are looking into the far distance and when you are looking at something at reading distance. In the latter case, the optician should allow for the fact that, because the lines along which you are looking are converging, the proper distance between the centres of the lenses in your reading glasses will be less than the distance between your pupils.

Of course, the stronger the lenses in your glasses, the more important correct centring becomes. In people who have had cataract surgery, without lens implants, and who rely on glasses, an error of an eighth of an inch in the centring can cause severe problems. I have seen patients who suffer constant double vision from this case and who are driven to desperation, just for want of a little more care in the proper centring of their glasses.

I would not like you to think that badly centred classes can permanently harm your eyes, however. They may cause symptoms of strain and, perhaps headache, and may damage your purse, but they will not damage your eyes.

Lenses that are too strong.
Another cause of spectacle intolerance is, regrettably, the prescription of excessively strong lenses for close

work. Inexperienced opticians sometimes yield to the demands of patients for glasses with which they can read the smallest print on the reading chart. Any patient who can be made to read half-way down the distance vision chart can easily be tried with progressively stronger glasses for neat work until the tiniest print can be read. But this may be possible only by the use of lenses which will force the patient to bring the print so near to the eyes that an intolerable degree of convergence will be needed. If there is a special requirement to see very fine detail, for work or hobbies, a special pair of glasses or a binocular loupe can be provided with the lenses deliberately decentred inwards to give a prismatic effect, so allowing the eyes to see together without excessive in-turning. It is important for older people to understand that an inability to read very small print even with their reading-glasses does not mean that there is something wrong either with the eyes or the glasses, but simply that they can no longer use accommodation and must rely wholly on the glasses to give them clear near vision at the focal length of the lenses.

Eyes with diferring refraction

Some people have the misfortune to have eyes which differ markedly from one another in their refraction. It is not uncommon for there to be a difference in the degree of long sight or short sight, and so long as the difference is minor, no trouble arises. But people with a large difference can be very difficult, or impossible, to suit with glasses. We call this condition "anisometropia", which is Greek for "not equal measure of sight" and it can be a real plague. This is because, although it may be quite easy to sharpen the vision of each eye separately (so that, when viewing with one eye at a time, the patient is delighted with the clarity of vision), this is done with lenses of very different magnification and the eyes see images of different size ("aniseikonia") which is very uncomfortable. The patient is not usually aware that the images differ in size, but may be acutely aware that something is wrong with the vision and that nothing is sharp.

So what is the optician to do? First, he must be aware of the problem and of its effects and must test the patient's reaction to simultaneous full correction in both eyes. Then he must see whether he can improve the patient's comfort by reducing the difference between the power of the lenses a little, even if this means less than perfect clarity in both eyes. In some cases, he may even, with the patient's full understanding and agreement, deliberately leave the vision in one eye uncorrected. Visual comfort is often to be preferred than visual clarity, and this is especially the case in people with a large difference in the degree of long or short sight. Unfortunately, many such patients can never be made entirely happy with their vision.

For completeness, I should mention that some people who have short sight in one eye and normal vision in the other, learn to use one eye for near and the other for distance vision. This is a particularly happy solution. Such people may never need glasses, either for reading or for distance, throughout their entire lives.

CHAPTER
TWO

Spots Before the Eyes

Every eye specialist is familiar with patients who complain of seeing specks floating in their field of vision. The symptom undoubtedly causes anxiety to a great many people, and the perception of these "floaters" has been around for a long time. The ancient Romans called them "muscae volitantes" (flying flies). There are even references to them in Chinese manuscripts dating back about 3000 years.

The experience of "floaters"

Concern about them can be deep-seated and sometimes difficult to dispel. I remembering once examining a rich American who, having retired from business, was spending his life touring the world with the prime object of consulting opthalmologists about his floaters.

The term "muscae volitantes" is quite a good one: often, these floaters dart about, very like small flies. I speak from personal experience. Floaters move with the movement of the eyes and, because the image of them is projected outwards, and the eye can move very rapidly, there is a kind of optical leverage which can make the floaters also seem to move very quickly. If you see one of these things to one side, and turn your eye to look at it, the effect is simply to move it, very rapidly, further away. This increases the illusion that one is seeing a small insect, and can be particularly annoying during reading — especially if one has the bad luck to have one right at, or near to, the point of gaze. Fortunately floaters seldom stay indefinitely in the same relative position, so one can be reasonably confident that a floater in this situation will, sooner or later, take itself off.

Floaters are best seen by looking at a plain, white, and very brightly illuminated surface, such as a wall on which the sun is shining, or at bright white clouds or even at a clear, bright sky. A man who was interested in this kind of thing once constructed a special room with a wall of white plaster, shaped like a hollow hemisphere, and intensely illuminated from behind the observer. Whoever went into the room could see nothing but the bright, white, curved surface, and immediately became aware of floaters. Many of these people had never experienced them before and some were quite alarmed.

Many people have noticed that their floaters are much more obvious, and numerous, on the morning after an evening of alcoholic indulgence. For this reason, the symptom used to be attributed to an alcoholic effect on the liver and they were even called "liver spots". I like to think of British officers in the Indian Army, sitting in their bungalows the morning after a night in the mess, gazing at the sun-washed walls, clutching their aching heads, worrying about their livers and swearing to give up brandy. I'm sure many of them were doing a great deal of harm to their livers, but that was certainly not the cause of the floaters. The real reason was a consequence of quite another effect of alcohol.

Alcohol is, among other things, a diuretic. This means that it increases the output of urine, in excess of the intake of fluid, leaving the body short of water and the individual thirsty. It also causes a concentration of the fluid within the eyes, so that there are more floaters within range of the inner back surface of each of the globes to cast shadows on the retinas. For that, indeed, is all that floaters are. We have been worrying about mere shadows. And because they are shadows we see them best when looking at something which evenly illuminates the inside of the eyes.

You can easily prove this to yourself. Find a situation in which you can see your floaters easily and fix your gaze on a point on the surface of whatever you are staring at. Look at this point, look away sharply, then look at it again holding your eyes perfectly steady. Your floaters will dart away and dart back again, but when your eyes are still you will notice that the floaters drift about, sometimes only slightly, sometimes a considerable distance. Now if these little specks were areas of disease on the retina, or any other fixed part of the eye, they would appear still when the eyes were still.

Floaters can take a variety of forms:

- Many are like little balls of fluff, rather out of focus.
- Some resemble tadpoles or spiders.
- Some resemble fine threads, or collections of cells.

One interesting fact about them is that when we see floaters, we are seeing structures which are sometimes so small that, if they were outside the eye, we would be able to see them only with the aid of a microscope. But, the nearer the object is to the eye, the larger it seems. In the case of floaters, although we cannot see a normal image of them (for they are inside the lens system) their shadows can be perceived, and because they are very close to the retina we can see their outlines even though they are microscopic.

Patients frequently expect me to see their floaters when I look inside their eyes as part of the routine examination, using an instrument called an ophthalmoscope to light up the inside while I look in. In the case of the common kind of floaters I have been describing, this is simply not possible, for the objects that are causing them are simply far too small. However, I shall deal, shortly, with another kind of floater which actually can be seen with an ophthalmoscope

Remains of tissue
What then, are these odd little bodies that cast their

shadows so annoyingly on our retinas? If you look at the eye diagram again you will notice that the greater part of the volume of the eyeball is filled with a transparent gell called the "vitreous" (meaning "like glass"). In fact, the vitreous is a remarkable structure and very important in ophthalmology. It consists of very nearly 100 per cent water, and what little solid matter it contains is very scantily distributed. The outer membrane is an extremely delicate structure of microscopically fine fibres of a substance called collagen — one of the main building materials of the body. But when the eye is at an early stage in its development the vitreous is more solid and contains some primitive blood vessels and other tissue. It is the remains of this tissue, lying on or near the back surface of the vitreous that throws shadows on the retina. Interestingly, because the vitreous is so fluid, movement of the eye in one direction causes the vitreous debris to move in the opposite direction. But because the shadow is cast on the part of the retina corresponding to the direction in which one is looking, the floater appears to have moved in the same direction as the eye. Fortunately, these remnants of developmental tissue are neither firmly nor permanently attached to any one part of the vitreous and frequently break loose from their temporary anchorage and drift away. This is why the pattern of one's floaters keeps changing, and why we need not be too upset if one happens to land just at the point of direct gaze.

Now I want to say something very important about floaters. As I have indicated, every one of us has them, although we are all not aware of them. They are normal, natural and of no medical consequence whatsoever. Although people experience floaters to different degrees, and indeed, some people have many more than others, the really significant factor is the mental attitude to them. I, myself, have hundreds of floaters and, being interested in such things, have observed them closely. Were I to concentrate on my floaters at all times, I would not be able to see anything else and would be quite disabled. But I would never dream of doing such a thing. When I concentrate on them I am very much aware of them, but when I ignore them I usually don't see them at all. Of course, if I happen to have one at or near the point of visual fixation, while I am reading, I find it annoying and difficult to ignore. But the last thing I would do in these circumstances would be to concentrate on the floater rather than on the print.

Unfortunately, some people, by their particular nature, are more prone to concentrate on the floaters than on what they should be seeing, and become progressively more disturbed by them. Such a one was my rich American. He knew perfectly well, having been told by a score of ophthalmologists, that his eyes were healthy and that floaters are of no significance, but he still could not ignore them. People who are so unfortunate as to be more concerned with the state of the functioning of their bodies than with using them to lead a full and satisfying life, are greatly to be sympathized with. Naturally, there should be a reasonable concern for one's health and well-being, but this should never overwhelm one's proper interest in, and concern for, the outside world and the people in it.

Spots of importance

It would be wrong to leave you with the impression that all "spots before the eyes" should be ignored. The kind of floater I have been describing should certainly be ignored, but it would be unwise to disregard dense, opaque floaters, and, particularly, those that genuinely interfere with vision. If you develop floaters (and if this happens, it is likely to happen suddenly) which actually blot out part of your field of vision, then the matter is one for an eye specialist. Such floaters might be coloured red, indicating that you have suffered a small bleed into the vitreous (a large haemorrhage into the vitreous blots out the vision altogether) and these small collections of blood often re-absorb and disappear. But, even if this happens, you should still seek medical advice, as it is important to find where the blood is coming from and, if necessary, do something about it. This is particularly important if you are diabetic, and such floaters should *never* be ignored.

A common cause of severe floaters but, happily, usually a temporary and unimportant one, is what eye specialists call "posterior vitreous detachment". As one gets older, the vitreous changes and tends to shrink. Because it is most firmly attached at the front of the inside of the eye, it tends to remain secure there but to come away at the back. In so doing it can cause quite alarming symptoms, including the seeing of a number of large floaters, sometimes red; bright flashes of light, which can often be caused at will, by moving the eyes quickly and, in rare cases, distortion or blurring of vision. All these effects can be caused by the vitreous peeling away from the sensitive retina behind, and if you experience them, you should seek specialist advise through your GP.

Fortunately, posterior vitreous detachment does not usually cause such severe effects, but it happens to almost all of us eventually. Although rare below the age of forty, it is estimated that about 60 per cent of people over the age of sixty have had a posterior vitreous detachment. Most of them will have noticed no more than a brief increase in their floaters and will be better off than before because, once the back face of the vitreous has come well forward of the retina (the space between simply fills with water), the debris in it is too far off to cast shadows.

There is another reason for reporting severe symptoms of the type I have described and that is that, very rarely, posterior vitreous detachment leads to a detachment of the retina itself. This is uncommon and very unlikely to happen but, if it does, it is a matter of the first importance for you. The subject of retinal detachment is dealt with in Chapter 9.

CHAPTER
THREE

Red Eyes

Surprisingly, when eyes look red, the redness is not in the eyeballs but in the thin, transparent membrane which covers the outside globe. This membrane is called the "conjunctiva" and is normally transparent, so that the white of the eye shows through. But it contains a network of tiny blood-vessels which, in perfect health, are too fine to be seen and it is when these blood-vessels enlarge, either temporarily or permanently, that the conjunctiva becomes red. The conjunctiva is firmly attached to the globe round the edge of the cornea and to the insides of the eyelids, but elsewhere it lies quite loosely on the eyeball so that the eye is able to move freely. If you pull down your lower lid you will see that the conjunctiva forms a connection between the globe of the eye and the lid. The same thing happens at the upper lid, but here the conjunctiva runs well back on the globe before folding forwards to line the upper lid. So the upper lid cul-de-sac is quite deep and people sometimes "lose" contact lenses up there, but it is impossible for anything to go right behind the globe.

The word conjunctiva comes from Latin, and

means "joined together". The ending "-itis" can be stuck on to the name of any tissue capable of being made red (inflamed) in this way, and one of the commonest known kinds of inflammation is conjunctivitis.

The conjunctiva is a very efficient, protective seal between the deeper parts of the ocular system and the outside world. But in serving this purpose it is exposed not only to the great variety of germs that inhabit our environment, but also to substances which can cause allergy, irritating dusts, fluids and aerosols, a variety of toxic or irritating gases and a wide range of forms of radiation. Fortunately, the conjunctiva is capable of replacing a good deal of the damage done to it, but if the assault upon it goes on too long, permanent changes — most obviously shown as redness — can result.

Infective conjunctivitis

This is sometimes called "pink eye" and is usually nothing much to worry about. It can be caused by any one of a very wide range of germs which usually get to the conjunctiva when we rub our eyes with our fingers. It is a fact that a considerable proportion of mankind knows little and cares less about personal hygiene and the effects the lack of it can have on others. So, wherever objects are commonly touched — in buses, trains and public places of all kinds, we must expect contamination. Any object handled in common may be a means of passing on infection; as, of course, may be direct contact.

Conjunctivitis starts with a feeling of irritation in the eye, associated with redness, usually in one corner. One may notice that the lashes are gummed with dried discharge and, especially on waking in the morning, they may be so stuck together that the lids cannot be separated until the discharge is washed off. A small quantity of pus may collect in the corner of the eye and there may be small blobs of yellow mucus in the tear film, especially down behind the lower lid. Soon the whole of the conjunctiva may be intensely inflamed and very red and if untreated the condition may spread to the other eye. Even if nothing is done, most cases of simple conjunctivitis will clear up within a week or two, but recovery will be more rapid if effective antibiotic eyedrops or ointment are used as early as possible.

Note that, although mucus or other discharge may get on to the cornea and momentarily obscure vision, conjunctivitis itself never affects the vision. If this happens, with a red eye, and you can't clear it by blinking, the matter is serious and specialist advice is needed. Similarly, although conjunctivitis may cause great discomfort, it never causes pain in the eye. If an inflamed eye is painful — either a severe, dull ache or a sharp pain, as from a grain of sand pressing on the eye — the trouble is likely to be more serious than conjunctivitis and, again, you need the attention of a doctor.

Not all forms of conjunctivitis will clear up in a week or so. Some fairly common virus infections can produce severe redness with swelling of the conjunctiva, and even of the lids, which may persist for several weeks and cause the victim much concern. But, however severe or persistent, if the condition is conjunctivitis, it will eventually improve.

I want to emphasize that any deterioration in vision, coming on rapidly in the presence of an inflamed eye, whether or not there is pain, is a matter of some urgency and you should not delay in seeking advice. An eye specialist, by examining your eyes with a special instrument called a slit-lamp microscope, will have little difficulty in discovering what is wrong and he will at once arrange appropriate treatment. Your GP seldom has the necessary equipment to do this and if you make it plain that your vision has been affected, he will appreciate the urgency and ensure that you are seen promptly by a specialist.

Some serious conditions

It is beyond the scope of this book to deal, in detail, with the more serious conditions associated with redness of the eyes, but a brief mention of some of them might be useful, if only to prompt you to seek advice without delay:

● Uveitis (formerly called "iritis" or "iridocyclitis") is an inflammation of the iris and the focusing muscle of the eye. The redness is worst near the cornea and there is nearly always pain in the eye and blurring vision.
● Corneal ulceration usually causes fairly severe redness but there is also a powerful awareness of a foreign body sensation, so that the person

concerned is usually convinced that there is something in the eye. If the ulcer is near the centre of the cornea, vision will be severely affected and the situation is grave, but if the ulcer is near the margin, and can be healed before it spreads inward, all will be well.

- An actual corneal foreign body, if very tiny, is unlikely to cause much redness, but a large one, or one of an irritating nature will do so. Such a foreign body should, however, be easily seen, so the cause of the trouble will be obvious, and it can be removed.

- Acute glaucoma is dealt with in a later chapter, but the symptoms are so severe that you are unlikely to be sitting around wondering whether or not you should do something about it. In acute congestive glaucoma, the eye is as red and as "hard as a brick", is agonizingly painful, and you will hardly be able to see at all. Fortunately, this is a very rare condition and there are usually preliminary warning signs, which you can read about in Chapter 7.

Sub-conjunctival haemorrhage

This condition sometimes looks alarming but, in fact, of all the many causes of red eye, it is the least deserving of worry, and I am glad to be able to relieve the anxiety it often causes. Sub-conjunctival haemorrhage is bleeding under the conjunctiva. The blood vessels of the conjunctiva are not only conspicuous, but are also somewhat less well supported than other vessels of the same size elsewhere in the body. It is by no means uncommon for vessels of this size to bleed spontaneously, but when they do so in other parts of the body, we are quite unaware of what has happened, because they are concealed. When conjunctival vessels bleed, however, the released blood spreads out behind the transparent conjunctiva to give a very conspicuous redness, sometimes in a localized patch, but other times extensively. You can distinguish this from a conjunctivitis by looking closely at the affected area and observing that it is not caused by dilated vessels but by a uniform patch of evenly distributed redness.

Sub-conjunctival haemorrhage is of no medical significance whatsoever. Some people worry that it might indicate high blood pressure, or a disturbance of the blood or disease of the blood vessels. In ninety-nine cases out of a hundred it means nothing of the sort. Often it follows a sneeze or a bout of heavy coughing and occasionally it occurs while one is staring at some physical task. But in the majority of cases it happens for no obvious reason. Repeated haemorrhages from the same point in the conjunctiva may indicate a minor local abnormality or weakness in one of the conjunctival vessels — such as a small varicosity (local enlargement and swelling of the vessel with weakness of the wall) but this, too, is of no consequence and easily dealt with, if necessary.

The blood under the conjunctiva begins to be absorbed almost as soon as it has been released and, usually, the evidence of haemorrhage has disappeared within about ten days. A very large one may take longer to go away, but sooner or later, all of them will disappear, and you should give the matter no further thought.

Chronic conjunctivitis

The word "chronic" is not well understood outside medical circles, and is usually thought to mean severe or annoying. In fact it simply means "long lasting". It comes from the Greek "chronos" meaning "time". So chronic conjunctivitis is simply conjunctivitis which stays with you. Conjunctivitis of this kind is not, however, the result of infection and has nothing to do with germs. Not all inflammation is infective in origin. It would be of advantage if it were because, nowadays, the great majority of infections can be cured, either by antibiotics or by the anti-viral agents available to doctors.

So why are some people's eyes constantly red? What causes the inflammation, in these cases? The redness caused by the enlargement and increase in number of the fine network of blood-vessels in the conjunctiva can be brought about in a number of ways, some of which are already familiar to us. The process of dilatation (enlargement) of these vessels is identical to what happens in the skin and, if dilatation of the skin vessels is allowed to go on for too long, they, too, will become permanently enlarged. A substance which commonly causes enlargement of blood vessels (vaso-dilation) is alcohol. The skin of the face, and especially of the nose may easily be flushed by alcohol and this state may eventually become chronic. The conjunctiva is no less prone to the vaso-dilating effect of alcohol and excessive drinking is one very common cause of chronic conjunctivitis.

It seems a shame, having got at the drinkers, to proceed at once to attack smokers, but there is no doubt that a common cause of red eyes is the chronic irritation caused by cigarette smoke, especially by retaining a lighted cigarette in the mouth. Many people become markedly sensitized to cigarette smoke so that merely to enter a room with a smoky atmosphere is enough to cause the eyes to smart and become inflamed. Although smoking is, unquestionably damaging to general health, especially to the respiratory and circulatory systems, I don't think it does much serious harm to the eyes, apart from tending to cause chronic conjunctivitis. Heavy smoking used to be believed to be a cause of a form of blindness called "tobacco amblyopia" but it is now known that this is primarily caused by associated heavy drinking, with severe nutritional deficiency. The arsenic in tobacco smoke can normally be removed from the body, but the absence of a particular vitamin (as a result of the fact that heavy drinkers often eat very little), interferes with this process of removal and the arsenic damages important fibres from the centre of the retina so that the victim has a large, central blind spot. Cure is easy, but as these people usually return to their former habits the long-term outlook is poor.

There is a skin and a conjunctival condition, a blushing disorder called rosacea, in which the eyes can become chronically inflamed; the fine conjunctival blood vessels can also extend on to the corneas and affect vision. Although rosacea is not very common, I mention it because it responds remarkably well to treatment if caught in time. Rosacea particularly affects the nose and the cheeks in a "butterfly" distribution and this characteristic appearance is easily recognized. Many patients with rosacea think that nothing can be done and put up with an embarrassing condition which could be relieved easily.

Exposure to natural elements

In some parts of the world, whole populations suffer from chronic conjunctivitis as a result of exposure to constant irritation from natural elements such as bright sunlight, wind and dust. This was very evident when I was working among the Arabs in Jerusalem. Almost every patient we operated upon had severe chronic conjunctivitis. Europeans who are exposed to tropical sunshine for long periods, may also develop a form of chronic conjunctivitis which is almost impossible to relieve. Certain wavelengths of the ultra-violet part of sunlight are markedly damaging both to the skin and conjunctiva and can cause permanent changes in the tissues. In the case of the conjunctiva, these include chronic enlargement of the vessels and thickening of the membrane so that a fatty swelling bulges forward on either side of the cornea. The person concerned suffers a persistent irritative discomfort with a feeling as if there is "sand in the eyes".

I would not like to suggest that there is major danger from the ultra-violet component of sunlight in a temperature country like Britain. But I suspect that the growing habit of deliberately exposing to bright sunlight, at every possible opportunity, as much of one's body surface as one's modesty permits, is likely to do more harm than good in the long run. The elastic collagen fibres of the skin, which give it much of its youthful quality, are damaged by sunlight and many of those whose chief concern has been the state of their physical beauty, have ended up considerably more wrinkled than they would have been, because of their determination to get a sun-tan at all costs. The same argument applies, with even greater force, to the eyes and, even in Britain, they should be protected from unnecessary prolonged exposure to the direct rays of the sun, especially in the middle of the day, when the ultra-violet radiation is most intense.

Other causes of persistent redness

There are several other local conditions which can cause chronic redness of the eyes, by inflaming the conjunctiva:

●   One of the commonest is blepharitis ("blepha-ron" is the Greek for eyelid). This persistent and annoying disorder of the lid margins is characterized by red rims, crusting, scaliness of the lashes and, in severe cases, even distortion and ulceration of the edges of the lids. It is not primarily an infective condition but is thought to be allergic in nature. It often starts in childhood and may persist throughout life. It is very difficult, if not impossible, to get rid of it altogether, but by proper treatment, it may be kept under control. Your GP will advise you.

Redness can be caused also by:

- Ingrowing lashes.
- Warts on the eyelids.
- Tear-drainage obstruction (see Chapter 4).
- Gout.
- Thyroid disease with eye involvement.
- Menstruation.

Fortunately, conjunctival inflammation associated with menstruation is rare, usually mild and occurs only from time to time.

Treatment

Many people with chronically red eyes are tempted to think that the solution lies in the use of eye-washes or eye drops. This is really an attempt to get rid of a symptom, and not good medical practice. Symptoms are warnings that something is wrong, and the correct approach is to discover the cause and remove it.

If the cause cannot be found, or has already lead to an irremediable situation, or if the sufferer is unwilling to deny himself the indulgence which is the actual cause, then some relief may be obtained by using eye-baths and bland eye-drops.

Your doctor can prescribe more effective remedies than those you can obtain over the chemist's counter but, unfortunately, not all of these are free from side-effects. Some, like steriod drops, although highly effective in relieving redness and discomfort, may sometime damage the eyes and therefore should be used with caution.

CHAPTER
FOUR

Watering Eyes

This is a simple matter to understand once you know a little about the system that keeps the front of the eyes wet and how tears are carried away. The minor amount of moisture needed to keep the corneas and the conjunctivas from drying (vision is impossible if the corneas dry) comes from a large number of very small tear glands in the conjunctivas. These glands continuously produce mucous which acts as a wetting agent, rather like a detergent, and salt water which forms a tear film. To prevent too rapid drying of the tear film a layer of oil, produced by other glands within the lids, forms the outer of the three layers of the tear film.

Excessive tears are not caused by overaction of these glands, but are produced by entirely separate glands which lie just under the bone at the outer and upper angle of the eye socket, on each side. These are the lacrimal glands and each is connected to the upper conjunctival cul-de-sac by a number of fine tubes down which the tear flows. It is the lacrimal glands that are at work when we weep or when anything irritates our eyes, such as a foreign body, onion vapour, strong winds, etc. Whenever the lacrimal glands function, salty water, sometimes in consider-able quantity, flows down the tear tubes and across the corneas. When these tears reach the inner corners of the eyes, flowing mainly along the gutter between the lid margins and the cornea, they arrive at two little holes, one in the lower and one in the upper lid and the the tears are sucked into these holes by an automatic blinking process. From each of these holes (called "puncta") the water passes along a fine tube into a small drainage reservoir (the "lacrimal sac") and, from there, down a much broader tube (the "naso-lacrimal duct") through the bone of the face, into the nose, fairly far back.

Now you know why the handkerchiefs come out during sentimental films. The sniffing and nose-blowing is due to an unusual quantity of salt water being released into the nose. If there were no outlet drain into the nose, these tears would flow over the lower lid margin as in weeping, and, indeed, if the rate of tear production exceeds the capacity of the tear drain, that is what happens.

Except in rare psychiatric conditions, emotional weeping does not occur continuously, but there are several other causes of over-activity of the lacrimal glands:

● Chronic conjunctivitis (see Chapter 3).
● Corneal ulceration or a corneal foreign body.
● Various allergic conditions of the conjunctiva.
● Poorly-fitting or dirty contact lenses.
● Exposure to a wide variety of chemical irritants dispersed as gases, dusts or fine sprays.

Commonest cause of watering eyes

But overaction of the lacrimal glands is by no means the commonest cause of watering eyes. The commonest cause of permanent, or very persistent watering, is a blockage of the tear drainage system. The watering that occurs as a result of this is called "epiphora" (Greek for "flowing beyond").

One very common cause of this problem is failure of the tear drain tube to open up at the time of its development. The naso-lacrimal duct begins, during the development of the baby, as a solid rod of cells running down from the eye to the nose. At or about the time of birth, the central part of this rod should have broken down and disappeared so that the rod became a tube. Unfortunately, if this process remains incomplete, there is an obstruction to the free passage of tears, and the baby will have a constantly watering eye.

A second consequence of the failure of canalization is that any germs which get to the eye and would normally be carried harmlessly away in the flow of tears, are not able to progress any further than the little lacrimal reservoir. So they accumulate in a spot which is ideal for germs to grow in: dark, warm, moist and protected. Thus, babies with epiphora almost always also suffer repeated attacks of infection in the lacrimal sac with the production of pus which oozes back along the small tear tubes to appear at the inner corner of the eye.

Sometimes the tear sac at the top of the naso-lacrimal duct becomes so filled with mucus and pus that it shows as a swelling on the upper part of the side of the nose. This condition should receive prompt attention, as otherwise the two small tear tubes coming from the eye may become blocked, an abscess may form in the tear sac and this may burst out through the skin to form a permanent opening. Every mother, whose baby has a watering eye, should be aware of the danger of allowing the lacrimal sac to fill up and, as a matter of routine, should gently press on the swelling or on the position of the sac — just below and inwards of the inner corner of the eye — twice a day. If the sac contains mucus or pus, this gentle pressure will squeeze the contents back along the two small tubes to appear at the inner corner of the eye. Keeping the sac empty in this way will prevent any real trouble. The method of sac pressure has another advantage. Usually, the naso-lacrimal duct is blocked by a fairly narrow and fragile obstruction. Finger pressure on the sac will exert a force on this tissue and, in about half the cases, will break it down and cure the problem.

In the meantime, however, infection should be kept under control by putting antibiotic drops into the eye daily. If the eye is still watering by the age of nine months or a year, specialist advice should be sought. The eye specialist will arrange for the child to be admitted to hospital where the obstruction can be broken down while the baby is under a short general anaesthetic. This takes about five minutes and is a very safe procedure. If it is not done reasonably early in life however, because of prolonged and repeated infection, the blockage is likely to become permanent.

Naso-lacrimal duct blockage is also the main cause of a permanent tendency to watering in adults, but in these cases the reason for the blockage is not so clear. No doubt a proportion of adults with this problem have had a blockage, or a partial blockage from childhood, but very few patients report a life-long history of eye watering. The trouble often starts intermittently and then becomes more constant. In such cases there is either swelling of the lining of the duct or temporary blockage with mucus or discharge. It is important to appreciate that, in many cases, matters have not proceeded too far at this stage and with reasonable luck, treatment can cure the watering. But this will not be available to you unless you see a specialist, so do report constant watering early.

Specialist treatment

If you do consult an eye specialist, he is likely to syringe the naso-lacrimal duct in an attempt to wash out any partially dried and obstructing mucus or pus. This is not a procedure to worry about. At the worst, you will experience fairly severe discomfort. You will probably be asked to lie down on a couch or a padded table while a drop of local anaesthetic is placed in your eye. This will sting quite sharply, but only for a moment. Then the tiny opening at the inner end of one of your lids, perhaps the upper one, will be enlarged with a small metal dilator shaped like a tiny pencil. This may cause you some discomfort, but the dilation of the opening is to allow the specialist to pass a smooth, round-tipped metal tube, called a cannula, along the narrow tear tube to the lacrimal sac.

The cannula is connected to a syringe full of a salt solution, and once the tip of the cannula is in the sac, the doctor will inject the saline solution along the cannula. This will cause you to have a slight, choking sensation as the salt water flows down the back of your nose, but there is no danger — simply try to remain relaxed and swallow steadily.

The slight choking sensation is actually a good sign, because it indicates that the tear duct is now clear and you should be free of further trouble. You will probably be given eye drops to use three of four times a day for a week or so. These are likely to contain an antibiotic, to keep infection at bay, and a steroid, to keep the lining membrane of the tear passages free from swelling. The doctor might insert a few drops of this mixture through the cannula, at the end of the procedure.

Regrettably, I have to say that syringing of the lacrimal passages, although effective in permanently relieving the watering, cannot be relied upon entirely for a permanent cure. In cases where the saline simply refuses to go down into the nose, it doesn't even give temporary relief and more radical measures are required, involving surgery, preferably under general anaesthesia, to make a new opening into the nose and to connect the the lacrimal sac to the membrane lining the nose. This involves making an half-inch wide hole through the bone, in an operation lasting for about an hour, and a certain amount of blood will be lost. If you have a large lacrimal sac, the specialist will find plenty of tissue to line the hole through into the nose and prevent it from closing by natural healing, and the operation is likely to be successful at once. But if the sac is small and shrunken, the doctor will probably feel it necessary to insert plastic tubes through the hole to keep the hole open until a natural lining has time to grow. This may take many months, during which it is possible that your eye will still water.

It is important that you should understand that you are not obliged to agree to such an operation. If you do not have it you will continue to have a watering eye, but no other harm will befall you. Indeed, there is sometimes a tendency for the watering to become less as time passes, so that you may be troubled only when out in cold and windy weather. If your main problem is a strong tendency to re-infection, as occurs frequently in babies, your doctor may agree to do a much smaller operation to remove the lacrimal sac. Many older people feel that they can live with their watering eyes and prefer not to undergo the major surgery.

CHAPTER
FIVE

Squints

A disadvantage of being an eye specialist is that one's attention is often attracted to people with squints and knowing how easily almost all of these squints can be straightened. I am sometimes tempted to open a conversation. But of course, that would be most improper, and so I remain silent. No such consideration need apply however, in print, and so I make the observation here. Although squints are not necessarily disfiguring, many squinting adults are distressed and have an unhappy awareness of the defect in the image they present to the world.

The main disadvantage of having a squint is that normal eye contact, in relations with others, is disturbed. One is not normally conscious of the importance of eye contact in conversation, or the amount of information conveyed in this way. Indeed, one need only think about the matter, while in conversation, to become aware of how disconcerting constant awareness could be. People with squints are constantly aware that those to whom they are talking are usually looking at the squinting eye, that is, the one not being used. So eye contact is lost and the relationship affected.

But cosmetic and social disadvantages are not the only effects of squint and, to make the whole matter clear, I will explain how squints come about and how important it is to detect and deal with them as early as possible.

A squint in childhood

At birth, babies' eyes are incapable of accurate alignment, but they should be able to move freely in any direction. If, a week or two after birth, the eye remains turned inwards and show no sign of outward movement, the matter should be reported, for the baby has suffered damage to the nerves connected to the small muscles which move the eyes outward. It is unlikely that the specialist would want to do anything surgical for several months — such cases sometimes recover on their own — but he will certainly keep the baby under close observation and will probably wish to operate at around eighteen months.

Babies born with squints may not have fixed eyes of this kind. Many have an inward turn of the eyes but are able to move the eyes freely and to use either eye to see with, whichever happens to be nearest to the object that interests them. But such babies can only use one eye at a time and, although the standard of vision is unlikely to be affected in either eye, they will never have "binocular vision", that is, the ability to see something simultaneously with both eyes so that it appears solid. Binocular vision never develops in babies born with squints, but as they have never had it, they don't miss it, unless they try to get a job in an occupation requiring it, such as stereoscopic photographic interpretation. Very few occupations require stereoscopic vision. When such babies have squint operations, this is done solely for cosmetic reasons, so there is no particular hurry and the child can safely be left to the age of three or four, when the anaesthetic risk will be negligible.

The cases which eye doctors really worry about are those in which babies born with normal eyes, develop normal binocular vision, and then develop a squint. You may recollect that, in Chapter 1, I explained that long-sighted children automatically focus their eyes in order to see clearly. Normally, this is done only when one is looking at something near. If something is close to our eyes and we are looking at it, the eyes must turn inwards if both are to be directed at the object. This is called convergence and happens automatically when we focus our eyes, under the control of a small computer in the stem of the brain. So, the two actions, of focusing and of converging the eyes, are closely linked and if you do one of them, there is a strong tendency for the other to occur also.

The commonest cause of squint
The commonest cause of squint, in young children, is long sightedness. Usually at the age when they are beginning to take an interest in picture books or small objects, for which fairly strong accommodation (focusing) is necessary, such children do so quite

unconsciously — but the eyes turn in more than is required. When this happens, the child experiences double vision, because, although one eye is looking at the object of interest, the other is directed at something else.

Now the juvenile brain has an amazing ability to adapt automatically to changing circumstances (an ability which largely disappears by the age of about eight) and the adaptation which occurs in a young child with double vision, is very rapid and takes the form of simply "switching off" the vision in the squinting eye. At the onset of the squint, these children screw up or shut one eye only. Squints of this kind do not develop in adults; the great majority of adults with squints developed them in childhood.

If an adult acquires a squint, either as a result of disease or injury, or the recurrence of a squint which started in childhood did not become fully established, the most obvious feature, to the person concerned, will be constant and uncontrollable double vision which will usually be so troublesome that he or she will cover one eye with a patch. At this age, there is no capacity to adapt by suppressing the vision in one eye, as happens in childhood. Long sightedness does not cause squint in adults. Squints starting in adult life are caused by damage to the brain or to the nerves controlling the eye-moving muscles, often as a result of head injury in traffic accidents, or, in the case of older people, from cerebral haemorrhage or thrombosis ("strokes").

Importance of early treatment

To return to the child who has just developed a squint and has adapted by turning off the squinting eye, let me make a very important point. If such a child is left untreated, there is no chance at all for normal vision in the squinting eye. The child will not complain for, at this age, children are unaware of the difference between monocular and binocular vision, so it is up to others to ensure that something is done, and done quickly. If your doctor says, "Don't worry, mother, he'll grow out of it," or "She's too young to do anything about it, now. Bring her back when she's older," insist on a second opinion. Otherwise, the child will be condemned to a lifetime of defective, perhaps severely defective, vision in one eye.

If caught early enough, squints caused by long sight can be cured simply by prescribing glasses of appropriate power to relieve the child of the necessity to focus more strongly than is normal. Indeed, a permanent squint will never develop and the child can grow up with normal vision in both eyes. But even if the squint is fully established, much may be done to reverse the situation, so long as the child is taken to a specialist at a reasonably early age. The eye doctor will start by checking the eye movements. If he is in doubt, he will inquire if either parent, or anyone in either family has or had a squint. He will also be interested in what happened at the time of the child's birth, and, in particular, whether there was prolongation of labour and whether forceps were used. He will ask many other questions and will examine the child, perhaps shining a torch at his or her eyes to see where the reflections fall on the corneas. He is likely to show the child some small, coloured toys and while the child is looking at these, he may cover the eyes one at a time.

The specialist will probably arrange for a test to determine whether the child needs glasses. This is not too difficult if, before doing the test, the child is made incapable of changing the focus of the eyes temporarily. This is done with a drug called atropine which, for just a few days, paralyses the focusing muscles which constrict the pupils, so these become very large. The ophthalmologist then uses a special kind of ophthalmoscope, in conjunction with a box of lenses, to find out the state of the child's refraction, whether long-sighted, short-sighted or astigmatic. If appropriate, he will then prescribe glasses and instruct that they should be worn at all times.

The specialist will then probably pass the case on, for the time being, to an orthoptist, an assistant who specializes in the management of squint. The orthoptist will examine the child with and without glasses, to check whether they are controlling the squint and will try to get a measure of the standard of the vision in each eye. If, as is very likely, the vision is found to be reduced in the squinting eye, the orthoptist will immediately arrange for that eye to start to try to see, by simply covering up the normal eye. Of course, great care will be taken not to interfere with the vision in the good eye by covering it for too prolonged a period. The child may well resent having its normal-sighted eye covered up and will try to remove the patch. So it is essential to ensure that the patching is, in fact, firmly stuck to the skin and difficult to remove.

It is my experience that indulgent parents often weakly give in to the child's repeated tendency to remove the patch. As a result the child continues using the straight eye and nothing is achieved. Success is often determined by the relationship between the parent and the child, but it is also important that the parent understands exactly what the surgeon and the orthoptist are trying to achieve. Fortunately, children who are confident of the affection of their parents will, when they see that their parents are determined, accept without protest that what they are told is necessary.

Perhaps you are wondering why I have never referred to a "lazy eye". This is not a medical phrase, and is not much liked by eye specialists as it rather suggests that exercises of the eye muscles concerned may cure the squint. It is true that the eye affected does not try to see, but the process is not so much "laziness" as a deliberate suppression of the perception. The poor vision in an eye with a squint is called "amblyopia" and this word is to be preferred as it has an agreed meaning.

Operation for squint

Quite often, even with proper management, and with full restoration of vision in the squinting eye by effective patching, the child still has a squint and the aim of the treatment to retain binocular vision, is threatened. It is at this stage that an operation to straighten the eyes is likely to be advised. This is done under general anaesthesia and takes about half to three-quarters of an hour. It involves opening the conjunctiva and readjusting the position of the connections of the small muscles which move the eye. In order to do this, the specialist will turn the eye strongly in the opposite direction. But there is no question of removing the eye as is often mistakenly believed. It is simply moved carefully to one side, to reveal the front ends of the muscles, and these are then detached and either sewn on again a little further back, or shortened to straighten the direction of gaze of the eye. The matter is a good deal simpler than might be imagined.

Most children seem little concerned or disturbed by the operation. Most are up and running about the ward early on the following morning, and seem indifferent to their temporarily swollen lids and inflamed conjunctivas, or they keep both eyes shut and stay in bed, sleeping, until more comfortable. Adult patients invariably make a great deal more fuss. I suspect that the basic difference lies in the fact that adults are aware, in some detail, of what has happened and are reacting emotionally to it, while the children are aware only of a fairly minor post-operation discomfort. The redness and swelling rapidly disappear and the eyes are usually white again in two or three weeks. There may be some reluctance to move the eyes fully for a few days, but this soon passes.

Surgery on adults

When surgery is to be carried out on an adult who has a long-term squint, one of the main concerns of the specialist is that he does not induce double vision. These patients hardly ever have the full binocular vision necessary to fuse the two images into one, but they may still be able to see, simultaneously, with both eyes. In such cases, so long as the squinting eye was directed well away from the object of interest, the image formed by it could usually be ignored. But if the eyes are straightened, the brain may not know which image to concentrate on, and the result may be double vision. Fortunately, tests can be done beforehand to assess the likelihood of this happening and if the surgeon advises against operation on these grounds it is best to accept his decision. Only once in such a case have I allowed myself to be persuaded, against my judgement, and I regretted it. In the end, after weeks of distress for the patient, to whom I could hardly say "I told you so!", I operated again to put the squint back.

Even so, I have always considered that eye surgeons should take seriously requests from adults for squint operations, even if for purely cosmetic reasons. To refuse to do so, simply because there will be no improvement in visual function, ignores the primary purpose of medicine, that is, to relieve human distress and, if possible, to add to the sum of human happiness. Resources are, of course, scarce, and some surgeons, short of operating time, may think that their time is better spent doing cataract operations to restore vision to the near-blind. There is also the concern that patients who also have personality defects, may believe that their problems stem from the squint and that all that is needed to promote their complete happiness, is to get their eyes straightened. Regrettably, this expectation is seldom realized and such patients may be worse off than before. The same principle applies to a proportion of patients seeking plastic surgery for real, or imagined, physical blemishes.

CHAPTER
SIX

Cataract

There are probably more mistaken ideas about cataract than about almost any other eye problem and some of these misunderstandings add to the distress suffered by people who know, or suspect that they have cataract. So I am pleased to have the opportunity to explain the nature and significance of cataract and, in the process, to give comfort and encouragement to the concerned.

Let me deal with the common misconceptions. Cataract is *not* some kind of "skin" spreading over the eyes. Cataract never, by itself, causes total blindness. Ordinary cataract in the elderly is *not* hereditary. Cataract surgery is neither painful nor dangerous and is, nowadays, usually done under general anaesthesia. Thick, heavy glasses are *not* inevitable after cataract operations. And when older people with very poor vision, present themselves to any eye specialist, the specialist is delighted when he finds that they have cataract, because the condition is now so easily and effectively remediable, by a skilled surgeon, that he would rather find this to be the cause of the poor vision than almost any other condition.

Cataract has nothing to do with the cornea (the front lens of the eye); it is yet another disorder of the fine focusing crystalline lens, lying behind the iris. People do sometimes get white scars on the corneas, especially poor people in backward countries where corneal ulcers become repeatedly infected for want of elementary medical attention, but this is *not* cataract. White scars on the cornea are conspicuous and easily seen by others. Until at the very late stage at which the crystalline lens is completely white, cataract is not apparent to the external observer.

Causes of cataract

We know a great deal about the way in which cataracts can be caused by penetrating injury to the eye, by a severe, blunt concussive force, by a variety of chemical poisons or by exposure to radiation of various kinds, but we know very little about the causation of the ordinary, very common type of cataract which just simply comes with advancing age. We know exactly what happens within the lens, but in spite of a great deal of scientific research, we are largely ignorant of why it happens.

When I tell patients that lenses tend to turn white, in old age, in much the same way as the hair turns white, I am not being very scientific, but this explanation often seems to be acceptable. The lens matter, as I have already mentioned, is composed mainly of fine, transparent fibres of protein, packed tightly together. This protein can easily be made to change its chemical structure so that it becomes physically altered. A commonplace example of this is what happens to the "white" of a raw egg when the egg is boiled. The white is made of an almost pure protein called albumen. In its raw state the molecules of albumen are arranged in a regular pattern, just like the fibres in the human crystalline lens, and, because of this, the "white" is transparent But when the egg is boiled, the protein coagulates, the molecules become clumped up and irregular so that the light cannot pass through, and the transparency is lost.

In a similar way when cataract develops, the protein in the crystalline lens becomes coagulated so that the light cannot pass freely through and vision becomes impaired. Of course it doesn't happen by boiling, but the effect is the same. Boiling of the lenses would, indeed, cause cataract, however, and there are cases on record where people accidentally exposed at short range to very powerful radar transmissions suffered cataract as a result of internal heating caused by the microwaves.

The lenses are sensitive to all sorts of influences. I might mention that cataract can be caused before birth by German measles and a number of other diseases. It can also, rarely, be caused by diabetes in adolescence and, later in life, can be brought on earlier than is normal, by the same disease. It can be caused by various drugs; by severe malnutrition and by electric shock. Almost everyone, if they live long enough, will develop some degree of cataract. Almost everyone over the age of fifty has some loss of transparency of the lenses; this is normal. What matters is the extent and density of the lens opacities and the speed with which they progress. Some people continue for many years, or even indefinitely, with fairly obvious opacities while, in others, the opacities progress quite steadily so that, within a year, or even less, of their first noticing a change in vision, treatment is required. I come to the surgical management of cataract later in this chapter, but I will just mention here that it is not possible to reverse the coagulation of the lens protein.

Cataract is, however, entirely painless. There are no nerves in the lenses and nothing happens to them which could possibly cause pain. If pain is associated with cataract, it is due to some entirely different cause. Secondly, cataract is *always* of gradual onset and of slow progression. If there has been sudden loss of vision this is *not* due to cataract. Of course, the awarness that one is not seeing so well as before may come suddenly, but that is a different matter. The patient who wakes up one morning to find that he cannot see, is not suffering from cataract. In the type of cataract that occurs naturally in older people the changes in the lenses are always gradual.

Symptoms of cataract

If he is observant, one of the earliest signs to the patient may be a change in the appearance of colours, so that blues are seen to be less bright and yellows and oranges are accentuated. Many people do not notice this until colour values are restored to them after operation. Many times, I have been told by patients that they had forgotten what blue really looked like and are astonished at its brightness. Another fairly common early sign is a change in the focus of the eyes in the direction of short sight, so that a long-sighted person who previously needed glasses to see the TV clearly may find that he sees better without them, and later discovers that he can read without glasses, although distant vision has become blurred.

This short sight by no means happens in every case, but it is remarkably common. If the cataracts are of evenly distributed opacity, the short sight may be very apparent and for many months may be the only symptom. But if the coagulation is irregular, the main symptoms will be clouding of vision and annoyance from scattering of light, noticed most when driving at night. However, many patients with cataract notice neither of these effects but simply find that they cannot see as clearly as before and that vision becomes steadily worse. And that is really all there is to the symptoms of cataract:

- Change in colour values.
- Temporary short sight.
- Light scatter and deteriorating vision.

No matter how dense the lens opacity may become, cataract never causes total loss of perception of light. The light may be so scattered (as is light passing through frosted or opalescent glass) as to prevent any formed image from being perceived, but the light will still pass through the lenses and will be seen as a variable glow.

Treatment for cataract

Sometimes a cataract develops on one side only, or is very much more advanced in one eye than in the other. If this is the case, and the vision is still near normal in the other eye, it is likely that the specialist will be reluctant to do anything. There are several good reasons for this, not the least of which is that he probably already has so many patients on his waiting list with both eyes affected that he feels that someone who is still able to see normally has rather low priority. Vision with one eye only is very little less good than with two. From time to time one sees a patient with a one-sided cataract whose work is made dangerous by the loss of peripheral vision on the side of the lens opacity. Sometimes, with a very dense, white cataract, there is also a cosmetic problem which may be very distressing. From time to time , I have operated for such reasons, but only when I have considered the patient suitable either for a lens implant or a contact lens. It is out of the question to use glasses to restore the focus of a one-sided cataract. I will explain this later.

Drugs, eyedrops, diets or any other form of medication or treatment are of no value in the treatment of cataract. Once the protein is denatured, it is permanently changed and cannot be restored to transparency. People who advertise alleged cures for cataract or who write books suggesting that you may have better sight without glasses are, at best, ignorant or, at worst, unscrupulously profiting by other people's distress. There is no cure for cataract except to remove the opaque lenses and this can be done only by surgical operation. Happily, this is now one of the safest and most successful of all surgical operations and, given that the eye concerned is otherwise healthy, offers about a 95 per cent expectation of restored vision.

Importance of early diagnosis

If a patient consults an eye specialist at a late stage of cataract it may not be possible to see past the opaque lens in order to examine the retina. The doctor may not be sure therefore that there is no other cause of defective vision. Various tests can give some indication of the clarity of the viterous and the function of the retina, but doubt may remain and disappointment is possible. So there is much to be said for examination at a fairly early stage in the process when, with full dilatation of the pupils and the use of a special binocular ophthalmoscope, the doctor will be able to survey almost the whole of the inside of the eye and pronounce upon its health. Even when an eye has been found to be entirely normal, apart form cataract, other conditions can develop simultaneously with the progress of the lens opacities. But this is very rare. In general, if the eyes are found to be healthy at an early stage, the probability of success is very high.

The examination by the specialist will be very thorough for he does not want to offer surgery unless he can be fairly sure of success. It will include a test of vision and a trial of new glasses, a careful microscopic check of the corneas and the front segment of the eyes, and a measurement of the pressure in the eyes (see Chapter 7) in addition to the attempt to to see the insides of the backs of the eyes. If the cataracts are already dense he will check if the patient can tell from which direction a light is being shone, and he will try this from all possible directions. He may order X-rays or a special examination using ultrasound which can give a representation of the inside of the eye behind even a dense cataract, in order to check for possible conditions like retinal detachment or blood in the vitreous jelly. The specialist will also be interested in the patient's general health and will probably arrange a chest X-ray, a full blood count and and electrocardiogram. These investigations are primarily carried out to assess the safety of the proposed anaesthetic. Nowadays, most surgeons prefer to operate with general anaesthesia but, if the tests indicate that this would involve any danger, local anaesthesia may be used instead.

It is very important at this stage to discuss the options for correcting the severe blurring of vision that is caused by removal of the crystalline lens. If a lens is removed from any optical system, the system will not be able to form a sharp image of any external object until either the original lens is replaced or another added to the system. This applies as much to the human optical system as to any other. There is one exception to this rule, and that is the rare case where the patient was so short-sighted, before developing cataract, that removal of the lens brings the eye into focus, by actually removing unwanted power. Although quite uncommon, this is very gratifying for the patient who, after a life-time of wearing thick glasses, is now able to see clearly without any assistance.

Cataract spectacles

In Chapter 1, I explained the use of dioptres in measuring the power of sight, and that most glasses have a power of only a few dioptres. However, if the crystalline lens is removed from an eye of normal refraction, and an artificial lens put in its place, such a lens will have to be of about +19 dioptres. If a contact lens is used to bring the eye back into focus, it will be of about +14 dioptres and if spectacles are used, about +12 dioptres. The differences in power are caused because a lens becomes effectively stronger the further it is away from the centre of the system. So, to see clearly without any correction after a cataract operation, one must have had about 19 dioptres of short sight before developing the cataract — and this is quite uncommon.

Ten years ago, the great majority of people who had cataract surgery were given glasses to restore the focus of their eyes. These glasses usually had to be very strong — about +12 dioptres — so they were very thick and heavy. Probably the worst aspect of such strong lenses was the frightening enlargement of the image and confusing distortion at the edges of the field of vision, which they caused. Over the years, it has been a source of some distress to me to note the difficulties many patients have in adapting to glasses after cataract surgery. Almost all find it very difficult. Many experience severe unsteadiness and insecurity as a result of the initial inability to judge distances and to cope with the suddenness with which objects seem to jump in and out of the narrow field of clear vision. Understandably, this makes walking down stairs very difficult, and crossing roads can be a terrifying ordeal. Many have told me that they are happy in their glasses when they are sitting quietly reading or watching television, but that moving about can be a trial. Recent research has shown that these difficulties are aggravated by certain changes in the part of the nervous system that controls head movements in relation to balance, changes which affect almost all old people, as a matter of course.

I mention these problems for several reasons. First, because it is important that people in this situation should be aware that they are not alone and that everyone with cataract glasses goes through this period of adaptation. Secondly, I want them to know that adaptation *does* eventually occur. Thirdly, modern "Aspheric" spectacle lenses, designed by computer especially for people who have had cataract surgery, give a much wider field of clear vision than conventional glasses. Fourthly, contact lenses can give almost perfect vision and are now so comfortable that one is often unaware of their presence. Fifthly, there is a growing tendency to short-circuit the whole problem by inserting an artificial lens in the eye at the time of the operation.

Intra-ocular lenses

Whether or not to implant a lens at operation is one of the most important decisions to be made at the time of booking for surgery and it is one the consultant, or his assistant, will discuss carefully with you, explaining the advantages or disadvantages. I am aware that some patients feel that they are not given enough time to consider this very important matter and others are too shy to ask questions about issues that are worrying them. I hope that this section may enable all patients to form their ideas at leisure and with all the important facts at their disposal.

The first thing to understand is that, if all goes well, the visual results from a cataract operation with lens implant, are usually excellent. The clarity and quality of vision are likely to surprise you, and you may be able to read without glasses. If that is the case, you will have been made a little short-sighted and will need weak glasses for perfect distance vision. Alternatively, you may have perfect distance vision without glasses, but require normal glasses of about +2.50 dioptres for reading. In no case will you require the thick, heavy glasses which would be necessary if no implant were inserted. You may be wondering why the kind of refraction left after the operation, should be in any doubt. The reason is that, even with the most sophisticated equipment, it is very difficult to calculate beforehand precisely the power required in the lens which is to be inserted into your eye. The required power varies with the curvature of your cornea, the distance from the front to the back of the eye (the focal length) and the actual power and position of the cataractous lens which is to be removed. This latter cannot be directly measured and there is always the element of guesswork involved.

Regardless of all that, the visual results are markedly superior to those obtained with glasses and about the same as with contact lenses, but without the need to put on and take off the latter (a thought that usually provokes anxiety in older people — until they master the knack). There is a snag however. In the last ten years, at least a hundred different designs of intra-ocular lenses have been produced, most of them as a result of dissatisfaction with one or other aspect of previous lenses. To some extent, the insertion of a plastic lens inside someone's eye is still experimental — and it can, and does, go wrong sometimes. In about ninety cases out of a hundred, however, everything goes very well, and these patients tell all their friends how marvellous it is to have lens implants and advise them not to consider any alternative. In fact, millions of patients have now had lens implants and the great majority have done very well.

This situation has forced some eye surgeons, especially those in private practice, to go ahead with intra-ocular lenses a little faster than they have been quite happy about. ("If you don't put in implants, doctor, I'll go elsewhere.")

Understandably, the great concern for all specialists is to determine which of the great range of different types of lenses now available is best. There are three basic groups of intra-ocular lenses, with scores of designs for each — lenses which sit in the front chamber of the eye, in front of the iris; those which clip on to the iris by means of small plastic loops, with perhaps a stitch through the iris; and those which lie behind the iris, supported by plastic loops stuck behind the root of the iris or in the capsule of the lens, which may be deliberately left behind for this purpose.

There is still a great deal of controversy among eye surgeons, as to which is superior, with some very powerful and authoritative opinions being expressed for each group. So the matter is by no means resolved and there are still many surgeons who, in spite of the manifest advantages of intra-ocular lenses, and the strong pressure on them from patients, from colleagues and from the natural desire to be "up-to-date", still cannot find it in their consciences to advise patients to have implants.

Possible complications

So what can go wrong? Our main concern is for the health of the inner lining of the cornea. If this is damaged, either at the time of operation, or later, as a result of contact with an intra-ocular lens, the cornea may lose its transparency and the eye may become permanently blind.

Damage to the inner lining of the cornea at the time of operation may not show itself for months, or even years afterwards. This is because the cells which form the lining, and which act to keep the cornea clear, have no power of regeneration. They must last us throughout our lives and tend gradually to diminish in number as we get older. All surgeons are very aware of the importance of avoiding corneal lining damage when putting in the lens. Fortunately, recent advances in technique, and the use of a new protective jelly-like material, have made this much less likely to happen.

Because of the importance of avoiding corneal contact, the methods by which the lenses are supported in the eye have received a great deal of attention. But here we have a dilemma, for the more firmly the lenses are stuck in, the more likely the supports are to cause damage by sustained pressure, with consequent long-term complications. One of these complications is glaucoma, dealt with at length in Chapter 7.

The presence of a foreign body in the eye can cause uveitis, a chronic inflammation of the iris and of the focusing muscle. This inflammation can persist for months, causing deposition of cells and fibrous tissue on the lens and blocking up the internal drainage channels of the eye to cause secondary glaucoma. If the patient is very unlucky and treatment fails, it may even cause blindness. Again, I would emphasize that chronic uveitis is very uncommon; and normally, treatment is effective.

Lenses may accidentally dislocate backwards into the jelly of the eye (the vitreous), so that the optical effect of the lens is lost and glasses or a contact lens must be worn. Finally, in this catalogue of, happily rare, possible problems, I must mention that lenses sometimes cause recurrent bleeding within the eye, which can be hard to manage effectively.

Anyone who had read this far may have been thoroughly put off the idea of opting for lens implants. But that has certainly not been my intention. To put the matter in perspective, one *must* record that there is a small element of the gamble about every surgical procedure, whether undertaken electively in the hope of improving one's condition or quality of life, or for dire necessity. Few major surgical procedures offer as high as 90 per cent success rate and that is about what lens implantation offers today. An increasing number of patients have had implants in their eyes, without problems, for more than ten years now and there is little doubt that the design of modern lenses has improved and will go on improving. With the exception of certain types of patients, described below, I am inclined to recommend lens implantations, rather than to discourage patients.

In my opinion, you should not have a lens implant if:

- You have only one eye or only one potentially functioning eye.
- If there is any history of chronic corneal trouble, or, indeed, any history of major eye disorder, apart from cataract.
- You should particularly not have an implant if you have had a retinal detachment in either eye (see Chapter 9).
- You should not have an implant if the eye is very short-sighted.
- Finally, if you are under the age of sixty, you should ask your surgeon whether he thinks implants are likely to cause trouble during your life expectancy.

The operation

It is perfectly natural to feel rather nervous at the prospect of such an operation and those who feel squeamish need not read the remainder of this section, except to be assured that at no time will they be aware of what is happening and neither will they be aware of any pain, even if the operation is done under local anaesthesia. The faint-hearted can now skip to the section headed "Recovery".

You will be admitted to hospital the day before your operation so as to be checked by the anaesthetist and to get your bearings in the ward. About an hour before your operation you will have a small pre-med. injection to calm you and make you feel sleepy, and you will probably be wheeled to theatre in quite a pleasant frame of mind. If you are having a general anaesthetic, the anaesthetist will insert a fine needle into a vein, probably on the back of your hand, and before you know what has happened you will be waking up, back in the ward, with the operation completed and a pad and protective shield over your eye.

If you are having local anaesthesia, for reasons of safety, you will be given a normal pre-med., often just 10 mg. of valium, and will probably fall asleep naturally. The procedure starts with a small injection just in front of the bump of the ear, on the same side as the eye to be operated upon. Then a second injection is given into the skin of the lower lid and continued backwards, over the edge of the bone, and into the eye socket. You will feel almost nothing except that you will become aware that the eyelid is drooping and that you are hardly able to move the eye. Finally, more local anaesthetic will be administered under both lids, so that all feeling in them is lost. You will then be left in the company of a nurse, with plenty of time for the anaesthetic to take full effect.

The actual operation takes much the same course, whether under local or general anaesthesia. The surgeon will use a swab held in long forceps to wipe over the skin of your face and will then wrap your head in sterile towels, taking care not to touch your skin or hair with his hands. He will talk quietly to you, from time to time, just to make sure that you are all right, and it is likely that a nurse will sit by the operating table holding your hand. Many surgeons, at this stage, spend about five minutes gently massaging the eye through a swab, to reduce the bulk of the vitreous and make the operation safer. The operating table may also be tilted so that your feet are downwards — you will find that you are more comfortable like this.

The surgeon will then gently fix your eyelids open with light retractors, but you neither feel or see this, because the sensations of touch and pain have been abolished, as has the conduction of your optic nerve, for so long as the anaesthetic lasts (and we tend nowadays to use one which has a duration of about four hours).

The operating microscope is now swung across over your face and this incorporates a very bright co-axial light so that everything the surgeon needs to see, through the microscope, is brilliantly illuminated.

You may feel a little heat on your face, but the anaesthetic will prevent you from feeling the greater heat on and around the eye. The surgeon will now turn your eye downward, put in a stitch to hold it thus and make an incision around the upper border of the cornea so that he can gently lift the cornea, like a little lid and remove the cataractous lens. Of this you will feel nothing.

Your implant will be ready, in a small dish of salt solution, and the front of it will be covered with a special protective jelly before insertion, to ensure that there is no contact between the lens and the inside lining of the cornea. The surgeon will gently slide the lens into the eye, ensuring that it is precisely in the right position and securely held. Then all that remains to be done is to sew up the incision with amazingly fine suture material. The stitches, although minute, are remarkably strong, and no restrictions will be placed on your movements afterwards. The surgeon will probably complete the procedure by giving an injection of an antibiotic, underneath the lower part of the conjunctiva. Some ointment may then be put on to the eye and a pad and shield fixed in place with tape, and you will be taken back to the ward. The whole procedure will have taken about three-quarters of an hour.

Recovery
As soon as you have recovered from the anaesthetic, you will be invited to get out of bed and be encouraged to walk about, or, at least, to sit up in a chair. Very little, if any, restriction is placed on

activity, so long as it conforms to what is normal and reasonable for a person of the usual cataract age. Lying passively in bed, without good reason, is undesirable because of the risks of encouraging vein thrombosis or chest infection.

You will probably stay in hospital for about five days so that the consultant can examine the operated eye daily to ensure that all is well. By the end of this time, the risk of most of the post-operative complications will have passed and it will be safe for you to go home.

The necessity to lift up the corneal flap, in order to extract the cataract and insert the implant, causes a temporary reduction in the transparency of the cornea, in most patients, so it will usually be several days before vision begins to return. But this is a very variable factor and some patients are amazed at the quality of their vision even on the day after the operation. However, it is important to understand that there are several reasons why there may be delay before the vision is restored, and you need not be alarmed or depressed if you do not see immediately:

● There may have been a tiny leakage of blood into the front chamber of the eye. This will severely diminish vision but is nearly always absorbed quite rapidly.
● Sometimes there is a delay in recovery of the normal tension in the globe and, occasionally, the front chamber of the eye remains a little shallow.

But these complications are uncommon and usually

resolve spontaneously in quite a short time. During the few days you spend in hospital, the nurses will put drops in your eyes three or four times a day and, when you go home, you will probably be asked to continue to use them. Do make sure that you understand exactly how to put them in — the nurses will show you, before you go. You should follow the specialist's advice closely, but if you do unavoidably happen to miss the occasional drop, there is no cause to worry.

If you have an implant, there is really nothing more to do but to wait for full restoration of the corneal transparency and full healing of the incision. The surgeon will not prescribe glasses until about ten weeks after the operation, because up to that time, the incision will be tightening as the scar tissue matures, and slight changes in the curvature of the cornea will alter the refraction. While you are waiting, you may find that your old reading glasses enable you to read with reasonable ease and there is no harm, whatsoever, in using them. For safety, I like my patients to wear a perforated plastic eye-shield for about two weeks after the operation, but at the end of that time I have no objection to their reading, or watching television, if they can.

If you have not had an implant, do not expect the vision to return to normal until you get glasses or a contact lens. However, you will be able to see, indeed, things may look extremely bright — and colours especially so. You will see outlines of all objects, very blurred but sufficiently for you to be able to get around safely. Possibly you may be given a pair of plastic glasses, called "temps", to use until your own glasses can be prescribed. Temps do have an approximation to the required power and are sometimes bifocal, but they are not intended to be accurate, so don't be unduly disappointed with the quality of vision using these. Some people like them, some don't. I remember one retired fishmonger who was so delighted with the vision through his temps that he refused to have anything else and was still wearing them when he came in for his annual check-up, complete with a present of dressed crab!

Contact lenses for cataract patients

With contact lenses, patients who have not had an implant, can still enjoy an amazing standard of vision and I always encourage such patients to try them. After cataract surgery, the sensation on the cornea is markedly reduced and, as older people have lax lids, their pressure on the contact lens is less, so the standard of comfort is usually remarkable. The only problem is that people who have had cataract surgery usually feel very unhappy about their ability to insert and remove the lenses, but many learn to handle them very well. One or two, however, rely on husbands or wives to insert and remove the lenses for them and the spouses soon become experts — putting a contact lens on someone else's eye is extremely easy, as is removing one.

CHAPTER
SEVEN

Glaucoma

You may have wondered how it is that a structure like the eyeball, which is essentially made of soft, collapsible material, not only maintains its shape but even retains a considerable degree of firmness. For the eye to function as a precision optical instrument, it is essential that the distance from the lens system to the focal plane (in this case, the retina, on which the image formed by the lenses falls) should be kept constant. The outer coat of the eyeball, consisting of the frontal cornea and the surrounding sclera, is remarkably strong, but has little or no rigidity. After death, the eyes become quite soft and are easily indented.

So it is clear that some active process maintains the firmness and shape of the eyeball. In fact, this is done in quite a remarkable way. Throughout life, water known as the "aqueous humour" is constantly produced within the eye by filtration from the blood and is forced into the interior of the globe to maintain its tension. This water is about 99.9 per cent pure and passes into the eye through the inner lining of the focusing muscle ring, just behind the back surface of the root of the iris. Have another look at the diagram facing page 1 to remind you. Aqueous humour should not be confused with tears. tears remain entirely external to the eyeball and contain a good deal of salt. Aqueous is formed *within* the eyeball.

Intra-ocular pressure

Perhaps you are wondering why, if aqueous is produced constantly, the pressure in the eye does not continue to rise until it bursts. This very good question is central to the issue of glaucoma. The whole of the main rear cavity of the eyeball is filled with the vitreous humour. This leaves comparatively little room for the aqueous which, having filled up the narrow space behind the iris, passes through the pupil and fills the space between the front of the iris and the back of the cornea. This space, known as the "anterior chamber" (front chamber) tapers to an angle just behind the edge of the cornea. This angle of the anterior chamber is the most important part of the eye, so far as glaucoma is concerned.

At the narrowest part of the angle, all the way round, is an outlet filter through which the aqueous gets out of the eye and returns to the bloodstream by way of the small veins in the sclera, near the corneal margin. So we have a continual process in which the rate of production of aqueous is balanced exactly by the rate of loss from the eye. Because of the resistance which the filter offers to the outflow of aqueous, the pressure in the eye is just sufficient to keep the globe nicely distended. And, because all the spaces within the eyeball are in continuity with each other, the pressure is even within the globe.

Now the inner structure of the eye — and in particular, the retina and the start of the optic nerve — being of living tissue, have a considerable nutritional requirement. The glucose, oxygen and other substances, needed to keep these structures functioning and healthy, are brought into the eyeball by the bloodstream. So, within the eye, there are many small blood vessels, and these are branches of larger vessels outside the eye, which enter the globe from the back. The blood inside these small vessels, is under a certain pressure, but so are the fluids surrounding these vessels. Moreover, the walls of the small internal blood vessels are extremely elastic so that if the pressure on the outside rose higher than the pressure of blood within the vessel, the walls would at once collapse, cutting off the flow of blood.

If the pressure of the aqueous rises above the blood pressure, the blood supply to the nerves is cut off, nerve tissues die and the vision is lost. Fortunately, it is not usual for this to happen suddenly although, rarely, it can. Much more common is the situation in which, over the course of months or years, nerve tissue is slowly destroyed and, with it, the fields of vision. This is glaucoma — a disease due entirely to the physical effect of excess pressure of the water within the eye.

Cause of increased pressure
You may wonder whether the rise in aqueous pressure is due to an increased rate of production or

to a blockage of the filter. In fact, it is always the latter. Although it is possible, by drugs, to reduce the rate at which aqueous is produced, it seems that a rise in the rate of production never occurs. There are many ways in which the outflow of aqueous at the angle can be blocked, but the effect produced depends on whether the blockage is sudden or gradual. If, by some uncommon misfortune, the whole of the filtration angle were suddenly to be firmly closed, the pressure would quickly rise to the point where every blood vessel within the eye would be closed. This rare kind of sudden, acute glaucoma is a very serious matter. Because of the rapid rise of pressure, the tissues of the eye are stretched and there is severe pain. The cornea becomes cloudy and of a greenish tinge, hence the name "glaucoma" ("glaucos" being Greek for "sea green"). The eye is intensely inflamed and very hard, and vision is rapidly abolished. This "acute congestive glaucoma" requires urgent treatment to save the eye.

Chronic *simple* glaucoma, caused by a partial obstruction to the outflow, so that the pressure in the eye is only moderately higher than normal, causes no pain. The affected eye is not inflamed and there are no symptoms. The person concerned has no idea that there is anything wrong until, at a late stage in the disease, his vision becomes severely defective, with almost total loss of peripheral vision and possibly even total blindness in one eye.

Negative scotoma

It may seem highly unlikely that anyone could

progress to this stage without being aware that something was seriously wrong. But it is indeed so, and happens to thousands of people every year. Let me explain. In each field of vision, situated about 15 degrees to the outer side of the point at which we are looking, each of us has a substantial area which is blind because the light rays from it fall on a part of the retina which has no light-sensitive cells. This natural "blind spot" is the projection of the head of the optic nerve, which contains only conducting fibres and none of the sensitive "rods and cones", the photo-cells of the retina, which convert light into nerve impulses and enable us to see.

But the remarkable thing about the blind spots is that we are normally completely unaware of their existence. We are not aware that we are not seeing in these two areas. I would like to try to demonstrate this to you. Sit down about a yard away from a blank wall on which you have marked a small spot, exactly at eye level. Close or cover your left eye and gaze firmly at the spot. Now raise your right fore-finger about a foot in front of your face, so that the tip is on a level with the spot, and with your gaze still fixed on the spot move the finger slowly to the right. If your concentration is so good that you can avoid looking at your finger, but keep your gaze on the spot, I guarantee that you will find you have lost the tip of your finger. As soon as you move your eye, however, the finger-tip will reappear.

You will have observed what eye specialists call a "negative scotoma". The word scotoma ("scotos" is Greek for "dullness") simply means a blind spot, and a negative scotoma is a blind spot of which one is unaware. (A positive scotoma is an obvious dark or black spot or area.) The main reason why one is unaware of a negative scotoma is that one is never actually looking in that direction and one does not usually see what one is not looking at. This is why people can suffer extensive loss of the field of vision without being aware of it. Of course, as soon as the field loss extends into the area of straight ahead vision, the person concerned is more likely to notice that something is wrong. But even then, the complaint is seldom of a blind spot, but rather of difficulty in seeing things like golf balls or in reading. People with advanced simple glaucoma do not see dark clouds around the point at which they are looking. They just don't see, and usually discover, indirectly, that something is wrong. I remember a lady who, somewhat against her will, eventually came to see me because her husband was fed up with her constantly bumping into people in busy shopping areas. "I don't bump into them!" she explained. "They bump into me, and I never see them until they do." Examination showed that she had hardly any peripheral field of vision. Fortunately, her central vision had not yet been affected and it was possible to save that by treatment.

Diagnosis of glaucoma

So, the important message about glaucoma is that it is quite easy to have it without knowing that you have it and that if it is to be diagnosed, one must look for it. Fortunately, knowledge about glaucoma is spreading and, indeed, one of my reasons for writing this book is to help to make the importance of the condition more widely known. I am delighted to be able to record that considerable numbers of opticians now carry out a glaucoma check as part of the normal eye test. Many early and treatable cases have been detected in this way. Like all ophthalmologists, as a result of such tests I am seeing more and more patients with treatable glaucoma. We are all acutely aware of the problem and every eye examination, however routine, includes a measure of the intra-ocular pressure.

Chronic simple glaucoma is rare in young people, but becomes commoner as age advances. At the age of forty, about one person in a hundred will have glaucoma; at the age of seventy, about one in ten will have eye pressures significantly above normal. Not all of these, of course, will suffer major field defects or blindness. However, very large numbers of people are blinded by the disease and it is one of the commonest causes of blind or "partially-sighted" registration in this country. Glaucoma runs in families and all relatives of patients with established glaucoma should be checked. Indeed, in an ideal world, everyone would be checked for glaucoma.

If you were successful with the demonstration of your own blind spots you can extend the method in order to carry out quite a useful, although necessarily crude, test of your own field of vision. To do this realistically, the eye not being tested must be properly covered and the eye under test must remain constantly fixed on a target of some kind. While gazing directly ahead at this fixed object, you should be able to see your outstretched hand round to the outer side almost 90 degrees. The visual field above, is naturally restricted by the bone ridge above the eye and by the eyebrow; in people with deep-set eyes it may be quite markedly restricted. The field below should extend down to the lap. The inner field is often considerably restricted, especially down and in, by the nose. I must emphasize that this is a crude test, unlikely to detect the curved scotomas, part of the way out from the centre, which are characteristic of glaucoma. Nevertheless it is better than nothing and if you wish, you may refine it by using smaller test objects than your hand. Please note that, although this is not primarily a test of the clarity of the vision, obvious differences in clarity in different parts of the fields are probably significant.

Specialist examination

If it is suspected that you may have glaucoma and you are refered to any eye specialist, you will have a full eye examination. In addition to testing your visual acuity, the specialist will be particularly interested in four things:

● Your intra-ocular pressures.
● The appearance of the drainage angles.
● The appearance of the head of your optical nerves (these are called the "optic discs" and often become hollowed out in glaucoma).
● Your visual fields.

Pressures are measured by an instrument called a tonometer which is used in conjunction with the ophthalmic microscope. You need not be alarmed by this. Although the instrument does press gently against your cornea, this will have been rendered totally insensitive by a drop of local anaesthetic and you will feel nothing. However, you must keep your eyes wide open while the test is being done, so that the eyelids stay out of the way. The head of the tonometer flattens a small area of the cornea to a standard extent, and the specialist notes the amount of force required to do this. This is a measure of the hardness of, and hence the pressure within, the eye. The same local anaesthetic drop allows the doctor to place on your cornea a kind of contact lens incorporating a small mirror, so that, with the microscope, he can look into the filtration angle of the eye and see whether there is any obvious cause of obstruction to the outflow. In chronic simple glaucoma the angle always looks normal, because the obstruction is in the internal part of the filter.

The optic disc is examined with an ophthalmoscope and the specialist will be particularly interested to detect any cupping, under-cutting or apparent loss of disc substance or displacement of the blood vessels which normally emerge from its centre. Cupping of the optic disc is not caused primarily by the force of increased pressure in the eye. We now know that all the small blood vessels which supply the optic nerve head are most susceptible to raised pressure and the first to get closed off. As a result, a proportion of the nerve fibres and some of the supporting tissue which, together, form the optic disc suffer atrophy and the disc loses substance. These nerve fibres, which originate all over the retina, come together at the disc to form a multi-way cable called the optic nerve, and it is damage to this cable that causes the defects in the field of vision characteristic of glaucoma.

These field defects can be studied with great sensitivity using special machines designed to detect them at a very early stage, and by repeated examination, it is possible to check that no deterioration is occurring. The consultant will put a patch over one of your eyes and ask you to fix your head on a chin and forehead rest while you look straight at a central point. Then tiny flashes or points of light are caused to appear at various positions on the field and your perception of them recorded. There are several different types of machine, some of extreme sophistication, involving computers and closed-circuit television. But don't worry. The more complex the machines, the easier for you to cooperate in the test.

When the examination is complete, the specialist will be able to tell you whether you do indeed have glaucoma, in which case he will also indicate the severity and explain the treatment that will be required. In most cases this involves no more than putting a drop in each eye twice a day and attending regularly for checks of the pressures and the fields. Most drops act by reducing the rate of production of aqueous, but some of them help to open up the drainage channels a little. Sometimes the basic eyedrops fail to control the pressures and various combinations or drops, and sometimes tablets, are required. In a small proportion of cases, even the most energetic medical treatment fails to keep the pressures below the upper limit of normal. In such cases, if the visual fields are progressively being lost, the surgeon has little alternative but to advise an operation to provide a new exit channel from the eye.

Sub-acute glaucoma

The acute congestive glaucoma I have just described, is really quite rare and occurs only if the outlet drainage filter is suddenly and totally blocked off. There is, however, a rather more common form of the condition in which the outlet channels are partially and intermittently obstructed and it is important that you should be aware of the symptoms of this also, for delay in obtaining treatment may be dangerous. This condition is called "sub-acute glaucoma" or "angle-closure glaucoma", and the rise in pressure occurs rapidly enough to produce quite striking, and very characteristic, symptoms which I will explain shortly.

Angle-closure glaucoma arises in people who happen to have eyes of a particular structural pattern in which the angle of the anterior chamber is naturally shallow. Such people are often hypermetropic, and as I explained in Chapter 1, hypermetropes have short eyes. I also explained that the crystalline lenses continue to secrete new fibres throughout life. In addition to making the lenses less elastic, this also makes them larger, and a glance at the eye diagram facing page 1 will show you that, in an eye with a narrow angle, increase in the size of the lens is not going to help. When the pupil is small, as in bright conditions, the iris will be nicely stretched out and thinned and the angle will be as wide as possible. But in such an eye, consider what happens when the pupil is dilated. Since the total bulk of the iris cannot change, if it becomes radially shorter, it must become thicker, and this fattening up may be sufficient to block off the angle, especially as the aqueous being formed behind the root of the iris tends to balloon it forwards.

This is why middle-aged, hypermetropic people with narrow angles, sometimes have problems when they go out at night in gloomy surroundings. For the patient, perhaps the most subtle and characteristic sign is that of seeing rainbow-coloured rings round lights at night. Now it is perfectly normal to see a yellowish glow around distant lights and, in rainy conditions, you may even see an occasional rainbow. But it is *not* normal consistently and repeatedly to see blue, green, orange, yellow and red concentric circles around lights. These "rainbow haloes" are caused by a quick rise in intra-ocular pressures which interferes with the insulating properties of the corneal lining so that tiny droplets of aqueous are able to pass into substance of the cornea from an anterior chamber. These droplets act on light rays passing through the cornea in exactly the same way as rain droplets act on rays of sunlight, breaking the white light into its component colours so as to produce a rainbow.

Rainbow haloes should never be ignored. They are an almost definite sign of sub-acute glaucoma or may, in rare cases, even be the first indication of an acute congestive glaucoma. Probably, they will be accompanied by other manifestations of fairly rapidly rising intra-ocular pressure. These are:

- Dull aching pain in, or around the eye.
- Mistiness of fogging of vision.
- In some cases, redness.

Of course, if a person having these symptoms moves into bright surroundings, the pupils will constrict and the angles will be opened again and for the time being, all will be well. Indeed, the best and the safest thing one can do in this situation, if at all possible, is to ensure that the pupils are kept constricted. Specialists will often use eye drops containing a drug called Pilocarpine, to keep the pupils as small as possible until something more permanent can be done about it. Incidentally, until a few years ago, Pilocarpine was the mainstay of treatment for chronic simple glaucoma also, because it often helps to open up the drainage angle. We now have better remedies for this, but Pilocarpine is still a most valuable drug in angle-closure glaucoma.

Repeated attacks of sub-acute glaucoma should not be allowed to happen because, every time part of the angle closes, there is the risk of adhesions occurring between the root of the iris and the back of the cornea. Such adhesions are serious as they progressively, and with increasing ease, block off the angle until, finally, total obstruction occurs. If these peripheral adhesions can be prevented the conditions can be treated by a simple surgical operation and a permanent cure effected. But if extensive adhesions form, the surgical treatment must be more radical.

Surgical treatment of glaucoma

Once a definite diagnosis of angle-closure glaucoma has been made, and examination of the angles with the contact lens mirror shows that adhesions are absent or minimal your specialist will advise you to have an operation. This entails making a small hole in the iris, near the root, so that the aqueous being secreted behind the iris simply passes through the hole and helps keep the iris back against the lens. This is a most effective and quite simple operation. Even if only one eye has been affected, the operation should be done on both eyes; otherwise, the second eye is likely to have the same problems. The procedure, called "peripheral iridectomy", is done through a small incision at the upper corneal margin, behind the upper lid.

For chronic simple glaucoma the operative procedure is called "trabeculectomy" and involves opening the conjunctiva and cutting a 5 mm square trapdoor in the white of the eye, just above the upper part of the corneal margin. This trapdoor actually involves only half the thickness of the sclera and when it is raised, a smaller square of the inner half, including a segment of the drainage channel —the "trabeculum" — is carefully cut out and a small portion of the iris is removed. The outer trapdoor is then smoothed back into place and secured with fine sutures. The conjunctiva is replaced and sutured to form a water-tight cover. The surplus aqueous is now able to leak out of the eye and accumulate under the conjunctiva, whence it is absorbed into the blood vessels. Thus, the pressure in the eye is prevented from rising too high. The results of this operation are, in general, excellent. But, in perhaps about one case in ten cases, it is unfortunately followed by gradual development of cataract. The latter is remediable, however, whereas visual loss of glaucoma is not.

The tragedy of glaucoma is that although its ill effects are easily preventable, thousands of people go blind, every year, from this well-understood and controllable condition. And, as the number of older people in our population continues to rise so will the number needlessly disabled in this way, unless something is done about it. Knowledge is everything.

CHAPTER
EIGHT

Headaches and the Eyes

The belief that headaches are commonly caused by some mysterious, and usually unspecified, defect of the eyes, is widespread and, I regret to say, is as very common cause of inappropriate referral to Eye Departments.

There are several reasons why the idea should have arisen that headaches are caused by eye disorder:

- The frequency with which headache is experienced in the region of the eyes — patients often complain of "pain behind the eyes".
- Each eye is surrounded, on three sides, by sinuses in the bones of the skull and if these are the site of inflammation, the consequent pain may be interpreted as coming from the eye.
- When a person has a headache from any cause, there is often increased sensitivity to light and particular discomfort in using the eyes.
- Migraine commonly causes quite major visual symptoms none of which have anything

whatsoever to do with the eye, as I shall explain later.

Some opticians insist that many headaches are caused by focusing errors in the eyes, especially astigmatism, and that these symptoms can be relieved only by the meticulous correction of even minor refractive error. This view frequently leads to changes of glasses, but I question whether it frequently leads to a cure of the headaches. The world is full of people with both major and minor refractive errors of all kinds, who have never been anywhere near an optician and who never have headaches. Refractive errors do not cause headaches.

Probably the commonest cause of headache is psychological stress, arising from one or more of the many frustrations to which we are all liable, and leading to a tensing of the muscles of the neck or face. Such persistent contraction has the same effects as over-prolonged use of any other group of muscles. If the muscles are not permitted to rest, recover and dispose of the waste products of their metabolism, they will soon begin to ache, and may even go into the spasm we call cramp. Certainly, one of the frustrations leading to persistent muscle contraction might be the inability to see properly to read, or to make out the print on a VDU, or to do one's job. And any of these difficulties may lead to a sense of strain around the eyes or even to aching in the muscles of the forehead or the eyelids. But in such a case, the origins of the trouble should be quite obvious.

As I have already indicated in Chapters 3 and 7, eye

pain can be a feature of inflammation within the eye or of a sudden rise in the pressure within the eye, but both of these conditions are accompanied by visual changes and are quite easily distinguishable from headache. This is pain due to organic disease, whereas the majority of headaches are due to excessively prolonged normal activity. Headache is, however, a very common symptom of neurosis, and the unfortunate people afflicted in this way often insist that their headaches are caused by an eye defect. A function as subjective as that of vision inevitably forms a focus of neurotic concern, and undue preoccupation with the process of seeing and a concentration on things like the normal variations, with age, in focusing capacity, the perception of floaters (see Chapter 2), and the resultant fear of blindness, will quickly give rise, in such people, to stress responses and neurotic headaches.

Migraine

Migraine is not well understood by the general public. The term is used quite loosely and is often incorrectly applied to ordinary headache. The word is a corruption of the Latin "hemicrania" meaning "half head" and one of the most striking features of true migraine is that it normally affects one half of the head only. In classical migraine, the sufferer often has a preliminary warning in the form of change in the general mood, sometimes to one of rising tension and irritability; sometimes, surprisingly, to a sense of well-being and energy. The "aura" as it is called can last for a few minutes or for hours and what may follow this is the reason for my including a brief account of migraine here.

Prior to the onset of severe headache — which is probably due to the dilatation and engorgement of blood vessels in the brain — there is often a phase in which part of the brain function is temporarily put out of action. Most doctors believe that this is because the arteries supplying blood to the relevant parts of the brain suffer a kind of spasm that severely reduces the flow of blood. Arterial spasm of this kind can most certainly occur, for the walls of the blood vessels contain circular muscles capable of doing this. This phase of the migraine may be very alarming to someone who has not experienced it before and who is unaware of the cause, for temporarily it may almost totally abolish half of the field of vision and the person concerned may think that he is going blind. Actually, migraine may cause a wide variety of transient neurological effects, even producing partial paralysis to one side of the body, but visual disturbances are by far the most common.

The visual disturbance usually starts as a small sparkling spot in the field of vision, usually to one side. This spot expands slowly, its edges being somewhat zig-zagged and scintillating and its centre being blind. Over the course of the next twenty minutes, and this time period is remarkably constant, the spot continues to enlarge until it occupies up to half of the visual field, and within that half field the sufferer sees nothing. A careful check will usually show that the field of vision is affected in both eyes, but that if the outer half of the field of one eye is involved, it will be the inner half of the other that is affected. This is called a "homonymous hemianopia". Such an effect cannot arise from an alteration in the function of the eyes themselves and, in fact, the eyes are not involved in any way. It is the part of the brain, right at the back — concerned with converting nerve impulses from the eyes into the experience of sight — that is temporarily out of action, and our detailed knowledge of the way the eyes are connected to this part of the brain fits in exactly with this half-field effect.

The same thing happens when someone has a severe stroke (cerebral thrombosis) affecting this part of the brain, except that the effect is usually permanent then, as the blood vessel has not simply gone into a temporary spasm, but has been permanently blocked. Similarly, the other neurological effects of migraine — paralysis, loss of sensation, speech upset, and so on, are all a temporary indication to the sufferer of what it is like to have a stroke.

As the effects pass off, blood vessels in the lining of the brain swell up and become engorged with blood. This is believed to be the cause of the headache and the headache can be effectively relieved by drugs such as ergot, which reduce the engorgement of these vessels. The hemi-cranial headache may be very severe and disabling, with acute sensitivity to light, so that the sufferer needs to lie down in a dark room. A constant feature of classical migraine is the severe nausea, and sometimes vomiting, that accompanies the headache. So the poor victim has a good deal to contend with and deserves our sympathy.

Migraine sufferers often worry that the effects they experience might persist. But of all the millions of people who suffer migraine, only a handful have permanent effects, so the chances of this happening are remote. Also the muscles that contract to keep the blood vessels in spasm can only continue to do this while they are supplied with blood. And in the action of closing off the vessel, they are actually cutting off their own blood supply, so providing a pretty good "fail-safe" mechanism.

Cluster headaches

I mentioned this uncommon form of migraine because it characteristically causes headache surrounding one eye and often makes the eye look very red. It usually affects young or middle-aged men, and the striking feature of the condition is that the headaches usually occur about once a day and in clusters lasting for from six weeks to two months. Each headache lasts for half to two hours and the interval between one cluster and the next may be months or even years. The headache may sometimes be present on waking but may occur at any time. The part of the head affected usually shows a striking flush of the skin, sometimes just around one eye, but sometimes affecting a wider area of the face or even the neck. When the eye is affected, the conjunctiva becomes very inflamed, because of engorgement of the blood vessels. The pain is often excruciating and, again, the sufferer may feel severely nauseated. There is severe sensitivity to bright light and to noise and the person concerned really just wants to go and lie down in the dark until the attack passes off.

It is important to understand that migraine, whatever form it may take, and whatever effects it may have, is *not* a disorder of the eyes. So treatment and investigation of migraine should not be delayed while time is wasted on pointless referral to an optician or to a specialist eye department. A great deal can be done both to prevent, and effectively treat, migraine, and special clinics and even national organizations exist to help sufferers get the best management. If migraine is your problem, you might wish to contact The Migraine Trust, 45 Great Ormond Street, London WC1N 3HD (Telephone 01-278 2676).

CHAPTER
NINE

Retinal Detachment

Retinal detachment is the one eye condition in which the signs are unmistakable. If you do get a detachment, you may or may not experience the preliminary symptoms (described in a moment), but what will certainly happen is this. A black curtain will appear in the field of vision of the affected eye, and, painlessly and unspectacularly, will progress like a straight or curved-edged, dark blind, totally obscuring that part of the visual field which it crosses. There will be no pain, no headache, just the dark curtain, which may come down from above, or up from below, or in from one or other side. Often, the appearance of the curtain is heralded by showers of bright sparks or flashes, sometimes followed by the appearance of many dark or dense floating spots, but sometimes there is no preliminary warning before the dark curtain is noticed.

Many people assume that retinal detachment invariably results from injury or blunt violence to the eye, but this is not the primary cause of the condition. Certainly, severe injury can, and does, give rise to detachment, and people who expose themselves to frequent blows to the head, as in boxing, must expect to suffer conditions like retinal detachment. But normally, the majority of detachments occur apparently spontaneously and quietly and often do so in people with apparently normal eyes, who have never suspected that anything was wrong.

Some people's eyes are, however, a good deal more prone to retinal detachment than others. Take another look at the eye diagram facing page 1. Since the retinal nerve fibres all converge to form the optic nerve, short of the most severe violence, there is no way that the retina can come adrift at the point where the optic nerve passes through the white of the eye. But elsewhere, the retina is not firmly attached to the underlying tissue, and separation is not difficult. Suppose, then, that the white of the eye expands for some reason, so that the volume of the globe increases. Clearly, unless the retina expands, too, there will be a very definite tendency for it to separate. As you already know, people with severe short sight (myopia) have eyes which expand to an abnormal degree, and they are considerably more liable to retinal detachment than people whose eyes are of normal size.

I must emphasize that, in those with minor degrees of short sight in healthy eyes (people with up to about 5 or 6 dioptres of myopia), the tendency to retinal detachment is no greater than in the general population. It is really only in higher degrees, where there is usually a good deal of degenerative change in the retinas and the underlying layer of blood-vessels, that detachment is relatively common. Even in high myopes, the condition is still quite uncommon, and the chances of any such person getting a detachment are probably no more than about one in a hundred. Of course, if you are a high myope and insist in engaging in activities like boxing, then the likelihood is much higher.

Fluid behind the retina

When the retinal detachment occurs in young people with apparently healthy eyes of normal refraction, the cause is often an unsuspected weakness in the forward attachment of the lower edge of the retina, sometimes associated with a small retinal cyst in that region. When the edge of the retina comes away like this, it leaves a large marginal gap and fluid from the vitreous passes behind the retina balloons it forward and then, progressively, strips it off, as the fluid works its way backwards. At first, the person concerned may notice nothing, but sooner or later, the curtain will begin to descend *from above*. Remember, the image on the retina is inverted, because light rays from above strike the lower retina, those from below strike the upper part, those from the right land on the left, and vice versa. I emphasize this fact, not simply as an interesting curiosity, but because it may be of major practical importance to anyone who gets a retinal detachment, as you will understand in a moment.

The business of fluid collection behind the retina is of prime importance and occurs in every case of detachment. In the very large majority of cases the process of detachment starts with the formation of a hole somewhere in the retina — usually peripherally, often in the area of degeneration — and usually the result of physical stresses. The tearing of the holes causes the light flashes and the dark floating spots arise mostly from haemorrhage from a small blood-vessel, involved in the tear. The shape of the tear often indicates the kind, and the direction, of the strain causing it. Once the hole has formed there is a strong tendency for fluid to collect behind the retina and soon, in many cases, there is detachment, with progressive ballooning forward of the retina. There is also the risk of further stripping off of the retina due to the weight of the fluid.

The vital part of the retina, for detailed vision as in reading, recognizing people, enjoying TV etc, is the central, very small area, we call "the macula". In glaucoma, we have seen that, so long as the macular area is not affected, the person concerned maybe unaware that anything is wrong, his peripheral visual loss being of the type we call a "negative scotoma". In retinal detachment, the peripheral visual field loss is very obvious. It is, in fact, a "positive scotoma". This is fortunate, for it tells us which part of the retina is detached and where the fluid lies, so we can position the patient's head to prevent further strip-ping off of the retina and, most important of all, *prevent the macula from being detached*. If detachment is confined to the peripheral retina, and this is put back again, the patient has an excellent chance of complete recovery of vision. But, if the macula comes off, he will never again have full vision and will probably have a very severe defect.

That is why it is important to know about the sub-retinal fluid and to understand that:

- If the black curtain comes down from *above*, this means that the retina (with the collection of fluid behind it), is detached *below*, and the patient should keep his head upright, or lie on his face. He must not lie down flat on his back until specialist help can be obtained — and this should be done as quickly as possible.
- Similarly, a patient with a curtain coming from the *left* side has a detachment of the right side of the retina and should lie on his right side.
- If a patient has a curtain coming up from *below*, he has a detachment of the upper part of the retina and should lie flat on his face, so that the fluid tends to track forwards.

Once the patient is in the correct position, the urgency is to arrange for him to be seen by an eye specialist. This is no case for waiting to obtain a GP's letter to a hospital. It is a matter for urgent referral after a confirmatory telephone call from the GP to the consultant.

So, what causes the black curtain? If the retina is to carry out its remarkable task of converting an image projected on to it into nerve impulses that the brain can process in order to provide us with vision, the light rays must pass perpendicularly into, and along, the light-sensitive cells (the rods and cones). Because the eyeball is spherical, in the normal situation, light rays always fall perpendicularly on the retina, even peripherally, and are able to stimulate these to produce nerve impulses. But if a segment of the retina is ballooned forward, the rays strike the rods and cones at a small angle and will not be directed along their length, so that they will not be stimulated to fire. In addition, a balloon area of retina will obscure flat and functioning retina, by cutting off the light rays to the latter. Most serious of all, the detached retina is now separated from its main source of nutrition, the underlying bed of blood vessels. Without oxygen, sugars, etc. it cannot function and, eventually, will lose the capacity to recover and will functionally die.

Examination for retinal detachment

If you have a retinal detachment, the specialist will have no difficulty in making the diagnosis, but to manage your case he will need to find the retinal hole. So he will put drops into both your eyes to widen the pupils and will ask you to lie down on a low examination couch. A very bright light proceeding from an instrument worn on his head, used in conjunction with a special lens held in his hand, will enable the consultant to get a very clear and extensive view of most of the inside of your eyes, while he directs you to look in various directions. The extreme edge of the retina is normally out of range even of this instrument, so he will gently indent your eyeball, mostly through the skin of the lids, so as to bring the extreme edge into view.

While carrying out his examination, the specialist

will make a sketch of the main features of the inside of your eye, on a special retinal chart. He will include the position of the largest blood vessels, the area detached, with reference to the depth of the detachment, and, in particular, the location, size and type of every hole present. The specialist knows that if he should fail to spot even one small hole, the subsequent operation to seal them off may fail to cure the detachment.

He also knows that it is important to carry out an equally thorough examination on the other eye, to see whether there are present any of the factors, such as retinal degenerations, or flat holes, which led to the detachment. If he should find anything of the sort, he will make another drawing as a guide and when operating on the eye with the detachment, will also seal off the affected areas in the second eye, to avoid further trouble. This is one of the most highly skilled processes in the whole of ophthalmology. An enormous amount of practice and experience is required to acquire real competence with the detailed examination of the inside of the eye, and to understand the significance of what is seen.

Operation for retinal detachment

The surgeon takes his drawings into theatre. The first thing he does, after the patient is anaesthetized, is to explore the sclera in the area of the detachment. The conjunctiva is cut all round the edge of the cornea and then along the appropriate line radially backwards, to give good exposure. Great skill and experience is required accurately to correlate the position on the outside of the eye, with the corresponding position of the retinal hole, inside. The difficulty is compounded, if the hole is at the apex of a retinal balloon. Correlation is essential to success, for the process of sealing off the hole, or holes, involved indenting the white of the eye from outside with a small sponge of silicon rubber foam and the minimal application of a device called a cryo-probe which actually freezes the tissues, right through to the inside. This must be applied in exactly the right area to cause an internal inflammation which will promote adhesion around the hole. The sponge is firmly stitched to the eye so that it causes quite a deep indentation on to which the detached retina settles and, because of the frost-damaged tissue, adheres.

This is how the majority of retinal detachment operations are done, but there are many in which much more radical surgery is required. It is now quite common for the surgeon to operate within the eye, using very fine instruments introduced through the sclera, a few millimetres from the corneal margin, and controlled by direct vision through an operating microscope used in conjunction with a strong contact lens.

In expert hands, almost all recent spontaneous detachments can be replaced and secured, and unless the macula has been off or has been affected by the close proximity of the edge of a detachment, the visual results are excellent. Most general ophthalmic surgeons see insufficient detachments to acquire the necessary level of expertise, and the trend is for a small number of interested surgeons to concentrate exclusively on retinal work, and provide referral facilities for the busy general men.

CHAPTER
TEN

Diabetes and the Eyes

By including a chapter on diabetes, I don't wish to suggest that people with this condition are exceptionally prone to eye problems. That is not the case. But diabetics do sometimes suffer undesirable changes in the eyes, directly as a result of the diabetes, and diabetes can affect the eyes in other ways. Some of these effects are trivial, but others can be of grave concern, so it is important that people with diabetes should be aware of the risks. Almost all of the eye complications of diabetes can be treated, usually with excellent results.

But let me put it all in perspective. Diabetes is an extremely common disorder from which millions of people suffer. The great majority of these never experience any eye complications at all, and of those who do, the majority are unaware of the fact and suffer no ill effects. But, although only a small proportion of diabetics are unlucky enough to have major eye effects from the disease, it is really essential that these people should know the facts, so that steps can be taken to minimize possibly serious consequences.

Rightly enough, diabetics tend to be concerned with things like diet, insulin dosage, how many Tolbutamide tablets to take, the levels of glucose in their blood and the output of sugar in their urine. They tend not to be aware of the fact that diabetes can have other effects, some of which arise from changes in small blood vessels in various parts of the body. It is as a result of these changes that the most important eye problems arise and I will come to them shortly. First I want to deal with some of the things that can happen to young diabetics.

Diabetes in the young

One eye effect of diabetes that often occurs before the patient is known to have diabetes is quite commonly the clue which leads to the diagnosis. I once worked in a hospital in which the Eye Outpatient Department was situated next-door to the Diabetic Clinic and there was a regular flow of patients from one clinic to the other. I think the younger physicians in the Diabetic Clinic were surprised at the regularity with which new patients sent through by the eye doctors, with a tentative diagnosis of diabetes, turned out to have the disease.

Examination of the eyes of these patients showed them to be entirely normal. They were young people who had had the same experience of becoming temporarily short-sighted. In some cases, by the time they were seen, the short sight had reverted to normal; in others, the focus of the eyes seemed to change from day to day. Now, as you will already know, from reading Chapter 1, ordinary short sight doesn't come on in a day. Nor, once present, does it ever disappear. So what could be the cause of these strange changes in the focus of the eyes of these young people?

Remember, the crystalline lenses within the eyes are readily able to change their shape so as to "accommodate" or adjust the eyes for close work. When thus accommodated, the eyes are temporarily short-sighted so that near objects are clearly seen. As you may have guessed, diabetes can alter the curvature of the crystalline lenses. If you are concerned with diabetes you will be aware that the disease is characterized by changes in the amount of glucose dissolved in the blood and the body tissue fluids. You will also know that, in untreated diabetes, the amount of glucose in a given volume of fluid can rise to dangerously high levels. This is not because glucose is, in itself, poisonous or otherwise undesirable. Indeed, glucose is the natural fuel required for the functioning of all human tissues. But too much glucose causes the tissue fluids, and the fluids within the individual cells, to act abnormally and to redistribute themselves abnormally between cells and the surrounding fluid, under the influence of a force known as "osmotic pressure".

An increase in the amount of glucose within the crystalline lenses will cause the lenses to swell so that their optical power increases. This is why the degree of short sight can be variable and why the condition can even revert to normal.

But any person who experiences periods in which

the distance vision is blurred but the near vision clear, or who has brief periods of obvious alteration in the focus of the eyes, should certainly not just shrug the shoulders and ignore it. At the very least, a test of the urine for the presence of sugar should be done. This simple test can be done in one minute by a GP. Normal urine contains no glucose, so the presence of sugar is almost always an indication that something is wrong.

It should be said that a patient who is having eye problems due to undiagnosed diabetes, is also very likely to be feeling unwell and will probably have noticed unusual thirst and a greater than normal output of urine. Symptoms of this kind should never be ignored.

People with diabetes are more prone to infection than others, and this applies particularly to skin infections such as boils and styes. Although not strictly an eye condition, styes are associated with the eyes and with diabetes. Both boils and styes are infections of the roots of hairs — in the case of styes, of the eye-lash roots. This is why styes cause "yellow-heads" on the margins of the eye-lids with a surrounding red swelling. They can often be cured by carefully pulling out the appropriate eyelash, thereby opening the small abscess and releasing the pus — a somewhat painful procedure, but a momentary one which may save the sufferer days of misery.

But this chapter is not really concerned with infection and my purpose in mentioning styes is merely to remind you that any person who suffers them repeatedly should certainly have a urine test for sugar.

Diabetic cataract

Diabetics are often worried about cataract and I am glad to have the opportunity to put right a common misunderstanding about this. Two kinds of cataract occur in diabetes and the one I am going to deal with in this section is, fortunately, very rare indeed. The other type of cataract, I will deal with later.

What specialists call *true* diabetic cataract is, and I repeat this for emphasis, very rare indeed. I have seen no more than a handful of cases of diabetic cataract in my entire experience, and I have seen many thousands of patients with ordinary cataract. This is fortunate, for it would be a devastating experience for a young person who may not even be aware that he or she has diabetes, suddenly, in the course of a day or two, or even a few hours, to find the vision misting out totally so that nothing can be seen but a white fog.

What seems to happen is change to the crystalline lenses of such severity that the capsules of the lenses become permeable to the water (aqueous humour) in which they are bathed, and millions of tiny bubbles of water congregate around the lens fibres, causing the lenses to become completely white and incapable of forming images on the patient's retinas. These patients are at once wholly disabled and it becomes a matter of urgency to treat them.

These patients are nearly always young — in their teens or early twenties — and the contents of the crystalline lenses are still very fluid. So the treatment is the standard operation for cataract in young people, in which the front capsule of the lens is opened and the contents removed. This is actually quite an easy operation and the results are excellent, but the young person is left with eyes which are grossly out of focus and have no ability to change the focus for different viewing distances. Contact lenses are by far the best way of dealing with the first of these problems, and reading glasses worn on top of the contact lenses will focus the eyes for close work.

Older people with diabetes do not seem particularly more likely to develop cataract than non-diabetics, but there *is* a difference. Unfortunately, on the whole, diabetics do tend to develop cataract at a somewhat earlier age than non-diabetics. This is purely statistical observation. Let us suppose that the average age of onset of visually disturbing symptoms from cataract in all persons is seventy-five (and this is just an estimate, as the age range is quite wide), then I think most specialists would agree that, in diabetics, the average age of onset would be from five to ten years earlier.

Here, I am referring to ordinary cataract of old age, not the rare, sudden-onset and rapidly-developing cataract. Cataract in diabetes is exactly the same as the ordinary cataract in the elderly, which I have described in Chapter 6 and there is really very little more to add. The treatment is exactly the same and the results of surgery, other things being equal, just as good. Because of their greater tendency to infection, diabetics who have had cataract surgery and who are wearing contact lenses should be particularly scrupulous about their standards of cleanliness in handling and storing the lenses.

Diabetic retinopathy

I have touched on this in Chapter 2, but would like to explain a little more about this important matter here. The term "retinopathy", like most medical terms, is quite simple when explained. The word-ending "-opathy" simply means "a disease of". Thus we have "myopathy", which is disease of muscle; "keratopathy", which is disease of the cornea; "psychopathy", a disease of the mind; "nephro-pathy", a disease of kidney, and so on.

The development of retinopathy is by no means a likely thing to happen to any particular diabetic. The fact that it is seen quite frequently by specialists is simply an indication of how very common diabetes is. And, even if retinopathy occurs, the probability is that the patient will be aware of no disadvantage.

Diabetic retinopathy is a result of the changes which occur in small blood vessels in the retinas, in diabetes and the commonest signs of retinopathy are tiny swellings in, and leakages from, these vessels. The swellings are called "micro-aneurysms"and appear, through the specialist's ophthalmoscope, as almost microscopic dark spots scattered about in the retinas. The leakage has two, apparently different, effects:

● To produce small blot-like haemorrhages in the substance of the retina. In this case, the leakage is of whole blood.

● The production of plaques of fatty material, called "hard exudates", in which case only the liquid component of the blood leaks out.

Both the haemorrhages and the exudates are, in this type of retinopathy, very small indeed and, fortunately, the parts of the retinas which we use for direct vision are often not affected. Indeed, the characteristic distribution of the fatty plaques often preserves the patient from any visual loss, as they normally occur in a circle around, but well away from, the important central area of the retina. Both types of leakages tend to be randomly scattered and it is very bad luck if a haemorrhage or a collection of exudates should happen to occur on the central retina.

Naturally, many attempts have been made to find a way of getting rid of fatty plaques, in the hope that those few unfortunate patients who have suffered visual loss from them may be helped. Regrettably, to date, none of these treatments have been successful. It seems that once an exudate has formed, the function of the retina underlying the exudate is lost. But research goes on and there is no saying what may be discovered.

A more serious type of retinopathy

A great many diabetics who develop retinopathy suffer no further ill-effects than the fairly harmless ones I have just described. But a small majority do suffer a more serious type and it is here that recent advances in treatment can be of great value. This form of retinopathy is called "proliferative diabetic retinopathy", and again it is a process involving the tiny blood vessels of the retina. But this time, in addition to the swellings, haemorrhages and hard plaque formations, something else happens.

It is as if the tissues of the retina were being insufficiently supplied with the vital oxygen brought by the blood, for, in these cases, new minute blood vessels grow from existing vessels and spread in fronds and networks over the surface of the retina. These new vessel networks would not do a great deal of harm were it not for the fact that vessels which bud out in this way are always very thin-walled, fragile, and prone to substantial bleeding. Here I am talking about bleeding which, in relation to the size of the structure within the eye, is sometimes quite massive. Such bleeding, occurring on the front surface of the retina, may spread over that surface. It may also pass forward into the jelly of the eye (vitreous humour). In either case, vision is likely to be affected, perhaps very seriously.

Repeated bleeding into the viterous is particularly serious. Often a small initial bleed will reabsorb and all will seem to be well. But then futher bleeding will tend to occur so that a tissue bridge forms between the new vessels on the retina and the blood clot in the viterous. This is a grave development, for the new vessels will begin to extend into the viterous cavity itself, further bleeding will occur, fibrous tissue will form and pull off the retina, leading to irremediable blindness.

Until a very few years ago, nothing which could be done to arrest or slow this terrible process. But today, we do have a means of combating proliferative diabetic retinopathy.

When proliferative retinopathy starts, it nearly always does so in a part of the retina which is very easily seen. You will remember that the million or so fibres from the retina all come together at one point at the back of the eye, to form the optic nerve. The fibres pass out of the globe through an oval hole and when we look at this area with the ophthalmoscope we see an oval pinkish structure, with some large blood vessels emerging from it. This is the head of the optic nerve, and is called the "optic disc". It is here that new vessels usually first make their appearance, and the appearance of these new vessels on and around the optic disc is something which must never be missed. Of course, unless they are looked for by someone skilled in the use of the ophthalmoscope and with the experience to know what he is seeing, the new vessels certainly will be missed and the measures now available for the control of proliferative retinopathy will not be provided.

Routine eye checks

For such reasons, it is now widely agreed by ophthalmologists that diabetics should have routine eye checks at intervals and that these checks should include the dilatation (enlargement) of the pupils with eye drops, and the careful examination of the retinas with the ophthalmoscope. Particular attention is paid to the optic disc and a deliberate search is made for new vessels.

What intervals are appropriate? Well, this depends on what is found at the first examination. Should the eyes be found to be entirely healthy, then they may probably be left for two years, but, should any diabetic complications be found, the interval would be much less than this. You can safely leave it to your specialist to advise you on this point.

If new vessels are found, before any bleeding has occurred or if bleeding has been minor, so that a view of the retina is still possible, the measure now available to us to minimize the risk of progression of the disease may be applied. The problem is one in which the tissues of the retina are unable to get a sufficient supply of oxygen from the existing blood supply. So one way of tackling it is to reduce the quantity of tissue competing for the limited blood supply. The retinas are very extensive and we make little use of the most peripheral parts, which form images only of what we see "out of the corners of our eyes". So we can, quite reasonably, sacrifice these relatively un-needed parts in the interests of the essential central areas of the retinas. If the peripheral parts of the retinas can be destroyed, or changed to "fibrous tissue"which has low oxygen needs, the limited available oxygen will be diverted to the central retinas which will no longer have the stimulus to bud out dangerous new vessels. Experience shows that if the peripheral retina is treated in this way, even established new vessels simply disappear! Moreover, they often do so in a matter of days.

There are several ways in which the peripheral parts of the retinas can be destroyed, but the safest and most convenient way is by the use of the Argon Laser and these expensive devices are now in constant use in most major eye departments.

I hope I have been able to provide the essential information about eye problems in diabetics without causing undue alarm. Let me repeat that major eye complications of diabetes are rare, but it is very much better to be safe than to be sorry. To remain in ignorance may, perhaps, be justified if there is nothing one can do to avert possible danger. But when remedy exists, it is important to know the facts.

CHAPTER
ELEVEN

Disciform
Degeneration

This final chapter deals with a condition which is becoming more and more common and for which, unhappily, in the present state of our knowledge, we can do very little. Disciform degeneration of the macula is a disease of old people. Like nearly all the diseases involving the back of the eye, it is entirely painless, often giving small indication of its presence until the vision has been severely damaged. It is slowly progressive and, tragically, often occurs in eyes that are also affected by cataract so that hopes of restoration of vision by operation may have to be dashed.

It is distressing, at the end of an examination of a patient with cataract, to find that the central vision cannot be brought back. I have never found it easy to explain to such patients that surgery will be of no avail and I find myself falling back on the somewhat doubtfully comforting assurance that they will never go blind. This is true in the sense that the condition affects only the central part of the retina and that "navigational" vision will be retained, but for the purposes of registration, these patients are legally blind.

To understand disciform degeneration one must appreciate that the macular area of the retina is free of retinal blood vessels and is dependent for its nutrition on diffusion of oxygen, sugars and other nutrients from the layer of blood vessels behind it. Between the retina and the blood vessels is an insulating membrane — rather like a layer of polythene sheeting — which allows the nutrients to diffuse forward but which, in health, acts as a barrier to the passage either of blood vessels or of tissue fluid. In disciform degeneration it as as if little cracks had developed in the polythene sheet so that fluid can seep through. This is the first stage in the development of the disciform and it is soon followed by the growth of fragile fronds of blood vessels through the cracks and these then spread out behind the macula. They also tend to bleed and, when this happens, a scar forms and, gradually, the whole of the central functioning retina — the only part we can use for straight-ahead detailed vision — is replaced by inert and non-functioning fibrous tissue.

Finding out about it

Major efforts have been made by research and clinical workers to find out as much as possible about this process, in the hope that some means may be found to prevent it. There seems to be some evidence that the development of the cracks is not simply the result of old age but may be an effect to which the person concerned is especially prone. It has been found that an early disciform can sometimes be arrested by using a laser to seal off the leaking spots. However, to use a laser to destroy tissue in the centre of the macula is simply to ensure blindness. So this method of treatment is of value only where the leaks are well off-centre, and this, unfortunately, is uncommon. Nevertheless, some people's central vision can be saved in this way, if the condition has not progressed too far. So it is important that older people should be alive to the possible significance of deteriorating central vision and should not ignore visual disturbance of any kind.

The initial leakage of fluid beneath the macula causes it to expand and to bulge a little forward. This produces a small area in the centre of the field of vision — precisely where one is looking — in which the image is reduced in size and out of focus. The perceptive patient may think that there is a shallow depression in the carpet or on the putting green. Later, as the macular changes progress, the central area of the field may appear distorted or may seem to have gaps in it. Reading may become difficult and as the damage extends to involve the whole of the macula, the area of visual loss increases until there is no useful vision within a circle of about 5 degrees around the point being looked at.

When the ophthalmologist examines the eye, at this stage, he sees that the macula has been replaced by an irregular, often whitish, raised plaque, sometimes with signs of bleeding into it, and he knows that there is no hope for the central vision of the eye. The only consolation is that the condition is, by its nature, restricted to the macular area so that the peripheral vision is preserved and the patient can get about with relative safety, although with very little satisfaction.

Registration of blindness

At this stage, the ophthalmologist will, as kindly as he can, suggest to the patient that the time has come for him to be registered either as legally "blind" or as "partially sighted". Once the idea has been accepted and the advantages explained, the patient will usually recognize that it is in his interests. If he does so, the consultant will complete the Certificate of registration, a form which contains all the relevant details of the patient's eye condition, and visual status, A person may be registered "blind" only if the vision is so defective that he is unable to perform any kind of work for which eyesight is essential. Anyone with a lesser degree of visual disablement but who is still substantially and permanently handicapped by defective vision, is registered as "partially sighted".

Registration as "blind" brings the following entitlements:

- An additional personal allowance for income tax purposes or a higher rate of supplementary benefit.
- A reduction in the cost of the TV licence and exemption from paying for a radio licence.
- Travel concession fares.

- Free postage on "articles for the blind" such as Braille clocks, specialized games, etc.
- Radio sets may be obtained through the Social Service Departments.
- Talking books are readily available from the Royal National Institute for the Blind (see below) or by taking out membership of the British Talking Book Service for the Blind, Mount Pleasant, Alperton, Wembley, Middlesex HA0 1RR. The annual rental will, in almost all cases, be met by the local authority.

Both "blind" and "partially sighted" registered people can enjoy a range of welfare services that local authorities are empowered to provide, and, after registration, a social visitor will call to explain the range of services available. These include:

- Assistance and instruction to aid in rehabilitation and the restoration of mobility and independence.
- Guide dogs may, in some cases, be provided. Information about this is available from The Guide Dogs for the Blind Association, 9-11 Park Street, Windsor, Berkshire.

The largest organization in the world concerned with the problems of the blind is the Royal National Institute for the Blind, 224 Great Portland Street, London W1N 6AA. They publish a catalogue of about 500 items specially designed for the blind, and sold by them. The RNIB also publishes a valuable pamphlet of information for people losing their sight and this contains full details of:

- How to go about getting yourself registered.
- What is available in terms of aids to rehabilitation, training and employment.

The RNIB also published a pamphlet on how best to relate to blind people and how to go about with them. It has a very large talking book library service and can offer a great deal of assistance with education, training, rehabilitation and recreation as well as advice and support for those seeking employment. Details of these and other services will be sent to you, upon application to the address given above.

Glossary

Accommodation The automatic process by which the focus of the eyes is changed when we look at objects at different distances. Very efficient in youth, but becomes progressively less so with advancing age (see *Presbyopia*).

Amblyopia A form of defective vision involving one eye only, and nearly always caused by a failure of development in childhood. After the age of about eight years the condition cannot be remedied.

Aniseikonia Difference in image size on the retinas.

Anisometropia Difference in the magnifying power of the two eyes. This causes *aniseikonia*.

Anterior chamber The front chamber of the eye, lying between the cornea and the iris. Filled with aqueous humour.

Antibiotic A drug that can kill infecting micro-organisms without damaging the patient. Antibiotic eye-drops are commonly used in infective conjunctivitis.

Aphakia The condition of an eye from which the crystalline lens has been removed, usually for cataract.

Aqueous humour, or "aqueous" The water which fills the anterior chamber.

Aspheric A special design of lens useful in spectacles for those who have had cataracts removed. The field of vision is greater and the distortions less than with normal spheric lenses.

Astigmatism The refractive error in which the cornea is more steeply curved in one meridian than in the other.

Atropine A drug dilates the pupil. The effect is prolonged. (See *Belladonna*.)

Belladonna "Deadly Nightshade" or "Atropa Belladonna". The active ingredient is atropine.

Bifocals Spectacles in which the main part of the lenses are used for distance vision and the lower segments for reading.

Blepharitis Inflammation of the margins of the eyelids. Tends to be very persistent or recurrent.

Cataract Opacification of the crystalline lenses.

Ciliary muscle The ring muscle which alters the tension on the crystalline lens to allow accommodation.

Conjunctiva The transparent membrane covering the white of the eye and lining the inside of the eyelids. (See *Conjunctivitis*.)

Conjunctivitis "Pink eye". Inflammation of the

conjunctiva. Commonly caused by infection with micro-organsims but also by many other things.

Cornea The front lens of the eye. Loss of transparency is a serious cause of defective vision.

Corneal curvature This, together with the length of the eyeball, largely determines the focus of the eye. (See *Refraction.*)

Crystalline lens The fine-focusing lens within the eye. Lies just behind the iris. Loses its elasticity with age and may become opaque later in life. (See *Cataract.*)

Diabetic retinopathy A disorder of the retina occurring in diabetes which, while often of little consequence, may have serious effects on vision. (See *Vitreous haemorrhage.*)

Dioptre The unit of lens power. The reciprocal of the focal length. A +1 dipotre lens will focus at 1 metre. A lens of +3 dioptres will focus at one third of a metre, and so on.

Diplopia Double vision.

Disc cupping Hollowing out of the optic disc. An important indication of possible glaucoma. Ophthalmologists always check the optic discs.

Disciform degeneration A disorder of the macula, leading to the loss of the central part of the visual field of the affected eye.

Endothelium The inner lining of the cornea.

Epiphora Watering eyes caused by blockage of the nasolacrimal duct. (See *Lacrimation.*)

Epithelium The important outer layer of the cornea.

Epithelial abrasion Damage to the epithelium by a scratch or by overwear of contact lenses. May lead to corneal ulcer.

"Floaters" Small spots which seem to be floating about in the fields of vision. (See *Muscae volitantes.*)

Glaucoma A condition in which the pressure of the fluid within the eyes is abnormally raised. Often unsuspected. The optic nerve can be damaged and scotomas caused. May lead to blindness.

Haloes Coloured "rainbow" rings seen around lights at night, in certain kinds of glaucoma. Should never be ignored.

Hypermetropia "Long sight". Usually unnoticed in youth, but becomes apparent as accommodation fails. Initially, near objects become blurred, then later the blurring extends to far-away objects.

Intra-ocular lens A plastic lens implanted in the eye after a removal of cataract. Three basic types. Gives much better vision than glasses, but complications sometimes arise.

Irido-cyclitis The same as uveitis. Inflammation of the iris and ciliary muscle. Usually quite serious and certainly calls for specialist treatment.

Iris The coloured diaphragm forming the back wall of the anterior chamber. (See *Pupil.*)

Keratoconus Conical cornea. Causes poor vision which can usually be much improved with hard contact lenses. May require corneal grafting.

Keratopathy Any disease of the cornea.

Lacrimal gland The source of tears in weeping or lacrimation.

Lacrimation Excessive production of tears as a result of emotion or irritation to the cornea or conjunctiva, or sometimes in internal eye disease. (See *Epiphora*).

Lacrimal sac The bag at the inner angle of each eye, into which tears run before passing down into the nose.

Lens A lentil-shaped piece of glass or plastic which is designed to focus light rays. The essential part of spectacles. The cornea is a lens.

Macular degeneration A range of diseases which damage the macula of the retina and cause loss of vision in the central area of the visual field. Usually untreatable.

Meibomian cyst A swelling in the thickness of the eyelid, caused by a retention of secretion in one of the Meibomian lid glands. Harmless, but annoying. Easily treated by a minor surgical operation.

Migraine A particular type of headache, usually affecting one side of the head only, and often causing temporary visual loss. (See *Scintillating scotoma.*)

Muscae volitantes "Flitting (or flying) flies". These

harmless floaters are caused by the perception of shadows of organic debris within the eyes.

Myopia "Short sight". Near objects can be seen easily, but distant objects appear blurred.

Naso-lacrimal duct The tube which carries tears from the lacrimal sac to the nose. Often fails to open in babies. This causes epiphora.

Ophthalmologist A medical practitioner specialising in diseases of the eyes.

Opthalmoscope An instrument for illuminating the inside of the eye so that it may be examined. There are several different kinds of ophthalmoscope with differing magnification and field of view.

Optic nerve The multi-way cable connecting each retina to the brain. Leaves the eye at the optic disc. The two optic nerves partially cross within the skull.

Optician (dispensing) A person trained to take frame measurements and arrange for the glazing of spectacles.

Optician (ophthalmic) A non-medical person, trained to carry out eye tests and prescribe glasses.

Orthopist A person trained in the management of strabismus or squint.

Pinguecula A fatty swelling in the conjunctiva on one or both sides of the cornea. Harmless, but may indicate excess exposure to ultra-violet light.

Presbyopia Literally, "Old man's vision". The result

of loss of accommodation. Reading glasses become necessary unless the subject is myopic.

Prism A wedge of glass which bends light rays so as to make an object appear to be in a different position from where it really is. Can be useful, in some cases of diplopia. Prism power is sometimes inadvertently produced in glasses by poor centering.

Pupil The circular hole in the centre of the iris. Varies in size with the brightness of the light.

Refraction The state of the focus of the eyes when the subject is not accommodating. Refraction may be myopic, hypermetropic, astigmatic, or emmetropic (normal).

Refraction error "Long sight", "short sight" or "astigmatism". Caused by a failure of proper correlation between the corneal curvature and the axial length of the eye, and usually corrected by glasses or contact lenses.

Retina The inner lining of the back of the eye. A photo-sensitive membrane on to which the image is projected by the cornea and the crystalline lens. The retina converts the image into a complex of nerve impulses which then pass along the optic nerve to the brain.

Retinal detachment Separation of part of the retina from the underlying layer. This results in complete loss of vision in part of the field of vision. The process is painless. Delay in reporting this is dangerous as all vision could be lost.

Rosacea A skin disease, associated with a tendency to blush, which can affect the corneas and damage them. There is an effective treatment.

Scintillating scotoma The temporary loss of vision in migraine. The edge of the blind area often has a sparkling quality called scintillation. The subject may see only half of the field of vision.

Squint The condition in which only one eye is directed at the object of interest. The other eye points elsewhere. Common in children and should be reported at once. Neglected squint, in children, often leads to amblyopia.

Strabismus Same as *squint.*

Tonometry The process of measuring the pressure of the fluids in the eye. The instrument used is called a tonometer.

Trabeculectomy The commonest operation for the treatment of glaucoma when the pressure cannot be controlled by eye drops.

Trifocals Spectacles with segments for middle-distance and near, as well as for distant viewing.

Uveitis Same as *Irido-cyclitis.*

Varilux lenses Spectacle lenses which provide progressively stronger power as the wearer looks down from the straight-ahead position. They are really multi-focal glasses but cause image distortion to the sides. Fitting and centring must be accurate. They are expensive.

Vitreous humour, or "vitreous" The jelly which fills the cavity at the back of the eye.

Index

ISIS

large print and audio books

If you have enjoyed reading this book, you will be pleased to know that many more titles are available.

We have listed a selection on the next few pages. These are available as large print books or unabridged audio books; some are available in both book and audio tape form.

Please write to us at the address below if you require further information or contact your local librarian.

Any suggestions you may have for new large print or audio titles will be very welcome.

ISIS, 55 St Thomas' Street, Oxford OX1 1JG, ENGLAND; tel. (0865) 250333

MEDICAL AND SELF HELP

	Longman Medical Dictionary
Christiaan Barnard	**Your Healthy Heart**
William H Bates	**Better Eyesight without Glasses**
Pat Blair	**Know Your Medicines**
Dr Robert Buckman	**I Don't Know What to Say**
Robert N Butler & Myrna I Butler	**Love and Sex After 40**
Margaret Ford	**'In Touch' at Home**
Margaret Hills	**Curing Arthritis**
Tony Lake	**Loneliness: Why it Happens and How To Overcome It**
Tony Lake	**Living with Grief**
Letts Retirement Guides	**Good Health**
Dr Patrick Mckeon	**Coping with Depression and Elation**
Dr Brice Pitt	**Making the Most of Middle Age**
Dr Tom Smith	**Living With High Blood Pressure**
Elaine Stritch	**Am I Blue? Living with Diabetes, and, Dammit, Having Fun**
George Target	**Your Arthritic Hip and You**
Dr Peter Tyrer	**How to Sleep Better**
Lynn Underwood	**One's Company**
Claire Weekes	**More Help for Your Nerves**
Betty Jane Wylie	**Beginnings**
Dr R M Youngson	**Stroke!**

ALSO AVAILABLE

	Longman English Dictionary
	Longman Medical Dictionary
	Longman Thesaurus
Lord Birkenhead (editor)	**John Betjeman's Early Poems**
Rabbi Lionel Blue	**Kitchen Blues**
Ian Botham & Peter Roebuck	**It Sort of Clicks**
Moyra Bremner	**Supertips to Make Life Easy**
Consumers Association	**Dealing with Household Emergencies**
Joan Duce	**I Remember, I Remember...** (Book and Audio)
Joan Duce	**Remember, If You Will...**
John P Eaton & Charles A Haas	**Titanic: Destination Disaster**
John Ebdon	**Ebdon's England**
Rose Elliot	**Your Very Good Health**
Margaret Ford	**'In Touch' at Home**
Leon Garfield	**Shakespeare Stories**
Ralph Glasser	**Growing Up in the Gorbals** (Audio)
Duff Hart-Davis	**Country Matters**
William R Hartston	**Teach Yourself Chess**
Stephen W Hawking	**A Brief History of Time**
Stanley Johnson	**Antarctica** (Audio)

ALSO AVAILABLE

Letts Retirement Guides **Finance**
Letts Retirement Guides **Good Health**
Letts Retirement Guides **House and Garden**
Letts Retirement Guides **Leisure and Travel**
C Day Lewis — **Sagittarius Rising** (Audio)
Jeanine McMullen — **My Small Country Living** (Audio)
Desmond Morris — **Catlore**
Desmond Morris — **Catwatching**
Desmond Morris — **Dogwatching**
Shiva Naipaul — **An Unfinished Journey**
Valerie Porter — **Faithful Companions**
Beryl Reid — **The Cat's Whiskers**
Beryl Reid — **Beryl, Food and Friends**
Sonia Roberts — **The Right Way to Keep Pet Birds**
Tim Severin — **The Jason Voyage** (Audio)
Ian Wilson — **Undiscovered**
June Whitfield — **Dogs' Tails**
Yorkshire TV — **Cooking For One or Two**
Andrew Young — **A Prospect of Flowers**

THRILLERS, CRIME AND ADVENTURE

Simon Brett	**Mrs, Presumed Dead** (Book and Audio)
Simon Brett	**A Nice Class of Corpse** (Book and Audio)
John Buchan	**Huntingtower**
Erskine Childers	**The Riddle of the Sands** (Audio)
Joseph Conrad	**The Secret Agent** (Book and Audio)
Peter Dickinson	**Hindsight** (Audio)
Peter Dickinson	**Perfect Gallows** (Book and Audio)
Colin Forbes	**Avalanche Express** (Audio)
John Gardner	**Icebreaker**
John Gardner	**No Deals Mr Bond**
John Gardner	**Scorpius**
B M Gill	**The Twelfth Juror** (Audio)
Paula Gosling	**Monkey Puzzle** (Audio)
Jeremiah Healy	**Swan Dive**
Patricia Highsmith	**Ripley Underground**
Patricia Highsmith	**The Talented Mr Ripley** (Book and Audio)
Elspeth Huxley	**The African Poison Murders**
Elspeth Huxley	**Murder on Safari**
Hammond Innes	**Campbell's Kingdom** (Audio)
M R James	**A Warning to the Curious** (Book and Audio)
H R F Keating	**The Body in the Billiard Room** (Book and Audio)
H R F Keating	**Dead on Time**

THRILLERS, CRIME AND ADVENTURE

H R F Keating	**Under a Monsoon Cloud** (Book and Audio)
Douglas Kiker	**Death at the Cut**
Deidre S Laiken	**Death Among Strangers**
Peter Lovesey	**Rough Cider** (Book and Audio)
Peter Lovesey	**Bertie and the Tinman**
Alistair MacLean	**Ice Station Zebra** (Audio)
A E Maxwell	**The Frog and the Scorpion**
A E Maxwell	**Gatsby's Vineyard**
A E Maxwell	**Just Enough Light to Kill**
Ralph McInerny	**Cause and Effect**
Brian Moore	**The Colour of Blood**
Marcia Muller	**Eye of the Storm**
J B Priestley	**The Shapes of Sleep**
Robert J Randisi (editor)	**An Eye for Justice**
Mary Shelley	**Frankenstein**
Patrick Süskind	**Perfume** (Book and Audio)
Dornford Yates	**Blood Royal**
Dornford Yates	**She Fell among Thieves**

INSPIRATIONAL

Rabbi Lionel Blue	**Kitchen Blues**
Victor Gollancz & Barbara Greene	**God of a Hundred Names**
Christopher Idle	**Famous Hymns and Their Stories**
Christopher Nolan	**Under the Eye of the Clock**
Beverley Parkin	**Say it With Flowers**
Beverley Parkin	**Flowers with Love**
Harry Secombe	**Highway**
	Your Favourite Songs of Praise

POETRY

Lord Birkenhead (editor)	**John Betjeman's Early Poems**
Joan Duce	**I Remember, I Remember...** (Book and Audio)
Joan Duce	**Remember, If You Will...**
Robert Louis Stevenson	**A Child's Garden of Verses**

HUMOUR

Ronnie Barker	**It's Hello From Him**
George Courtauld	**Odd Noises From the Barn**
John Ebdon	**Ebdon's England**
	Echoes of Laughter
Mary Dunn	**Lady Addle Remembers**
Joyce Fussey	**Cats in the Coffee**
Joyce Fussey	**'Milk My Ewes and Weep'**
George & Weedon Grossmith	**The Diary of a Nobody**
Maureen Lipman	**How Was It For You?**
Spike Milligan	**Adolf Hitler: My Part in His Downfall (Book and Audio)**
Spike Milligan	**Mussolini: His Part in My Downfall (Audio)**
Spike Milligan	**Rommel: Gunner Who? and Monty His Part in My Victory (Audio)**
Spike Milligan	**Where Have All the Bullets Gone? (Audio)**
Derek Nimmo	**Up Mount Everest Without a Paddle**
Barry Pain	**The Eliza Stories**
Walter Carruthers Sellar & Robert Julian Yeatman	**1066 and All That**
Tom Sharpe	**Blott on the Landscape**
Tom Sharpe	**Porterhouse Blue**
Tom Sharpe	**Vintage Stuff (Book and Audio)**
Tom Sharpe	**Wilt**
Tom Sharpe	**Wilt on High**
E OE Somerville & Martin Ross	**Further Experiences of an Irish RM,**
E OE Somerville & Martin Ross	**In Mr Knox's Country**

SHORT STORIES AND ESSAYS

	Echoes of Laughter
Jorges Louis Borges	**The Book of Sand**
Angela Carter	**Fireworks**
Joseph Conrad	**The Heart of Darkness** (Audio)
A E Coppard	**Selected Stories**
Roald Dahl	**Roald Dahl's Book of Ghost Stories**
Roald Dahl	**Kiss Kiss**
M F K Fisher	**Sister Age**
E M Forster	**The New Collected Short Stories** (Audio)
Jane Gardam	**The Sidmouth Letters**
Leon Garfield	**Shakespeare Stories**
Mrs Gaskell	**Four Short Stories**
William Golding	**The Hot Gates**
Thomas Hardy	**Wessex Tales**
Duff Hart-Davis	**Country Matters**
Henry James	**Daisy Miller**
M R James	**A Warning to the Curious** (Book and Audio)
Bernard Levin	**The Way We Live Now**
Barry Pain	**The Eliza Stories**
Robert J Randisi (editor)	**An Eye for Justice**
Saki	**Beasts and Superbeasts**
E OE Somerville & Martin Ross	**Further Experiences of an Irish RM**
E OE Somerville & Martin Ross	**In Mr Knox's Country**
Edmund Wilson	**Memoirs of Hecate County**
Marguerite Yourcenar	**Oriental Tales**